Percutaneous Approaches to Valvular Heart Disease

Guest Editors

SAMIN K. SHARMA, MD
IGOR F. PALACIOS, MD

INTERVENTIONAL CARDIOLOGY CLINICS

www.interventional.theclinics.com

Consulting Editors
SAMIN K. SHARMA, MD
IGOR F. PALACIOS, MD

January 2012 • Volume 1 • Number 1

SAUNDERS an imprint of ELSEVIER, Inc.

W.B. SAUNDERS COMPANY
A Division of Elsevier Inc.

1600 John F. Kennedy Boulevard • Suite 1800 • Philadelphia, Pennsylvania 19103-2899

http://www.theclinics.com

INTERVENTIONAL CARDIOLOGY CLINICS Volume 1, Number 1
January 2012 ISSN 2211-7458, ISBN-13: 978-1-4557-3881-6

Editor: Barbara Cohen-Kligerman
Developmental Editor: Teia Stone

Interventional Cardiology Clinics (ISSN 2211-7458) is published quarterly by Elsevier Inc., 360 Park Avenue South, New York, NY 10010-1710. Months of issue are January, April, July, and October. Subscription prices are USD 177 per year for US individuals, USD 119 per year for US students, USD 265 per year for Canadian individuals, USD 129 per year for Canadian students, USD 265 per year for international individuals, and USD 136 per year for international students. To receive student/resident rate, orders must be accompanied by name of affiliated institution, date of term, and the *signature* of program/residency coordinator on institution letterhead. Orders will be billed at individual rate until proof of status is received. Foreign air speed delivery is included in all *Clinics* subscription prices. All prices are subject to change without notice. **POSTMASTER:** Send address changes to *Interventional Cardiology Clinics*, Elsevier Health Sciences Division, Subscription Customer Service, 3251 Riverport Lane, Maryland Heights, MO 63043. **Customer Service: Telephone: 1-800-654-2452** (U.S. and Canada); **1-314-447-8871** (outside U.S. and Canada). **Fax: 1-314-447-8029. E-mail: journalscustomerservice-usa@elsevier.com** (for print support); **journalsonlinesupport-usa@elsevier.com** (for online support).

Reprints. For copies of 100 or more of articles in this publication, please contact the Commercial Reprints Department, Elsevier Inc., 360 Park Avenue South, New York, NY 10010-1710. Tel.: 212-633-3812; Fax: 212-462-1935; E-mail: reprints@elsevier.com.

Printed and bound by CPI Group (UK) Ltd, Croydon, CR0 4YY

Transferred to Digital Print 2012

Contributors

CONSULTING EDITORS

SAMIN K. SHARMA, MD, FSCAI, FACC
Director of Clinical Cardiology; Director of
Cardiac Catheterization Laboratory, Mount
Sinai Medical Center, New York, New York

IGOR F. PALACIOS, MD, FSCAI
Director of Interventional Cardiology,
Cardiology Division, Heart Center,
Massachusetts General Hospital; Associate
Professor of Medicine, Harvard Medical
School, Boston, Massachusetts

GUEST EDITORS

SAMIN K. SHARMA, MD, FSCAI, FACC
Director of Clinical Cardiology; Director of
Cardiac Catheterization Laboratory, Mount
Sinai Medical Center, New York, New York

IGOR F. PALACIOS, MD, FSCAI
Director of Interventional Cardiology,
Cardiology Division, Heart Center,
Massachusetts General Hospital; Associate
Professor of Medicine, Harvard Medical
School, Boston, Massachusetts

AUTHORS

DABIT ARZAMENDI, MD, MSc
Fellow in Interventional Cardiology and
Structural Heart Disease, Cardiology Division,
Massachusetts General Hospital, Harvard
Medical School, Boston Massachusetts

ANITA W. ASGAR, MD, FRCPC
Assistant Professor of Medicine, Université de
Montréal, Montreal, Canada

USMAN BABER, MD, MS
Director of Clinical Biometrics; Assistant
Professor of Medicine, Cardiac Catheterization
Laboratory, Mount Sinai Medical Center,
New York, New York

RAOUL BONAN, MD
Associate Professor of Medicine, University of
Montreal, Montreal, Canada

ALAIN CRIBIER, MD
Professor of Medicine, Department of
Cardiology, Charles Nicolle University Hospital,
Rouen, France

ROBERTO J. CUBEDDU, MD
Interventional Cardiology and Structural Heart
Disease, Massachusetts General Hospital,
Harvard Medical School, Boston,
Massachusetts

SAMMY ELMARIAH, MD, MPH
Fellow in Interventional Cardiology and
Structural Heart Disease, Cardiology Division,
Massachusetts General Hospital, Harvard
Medical School, Boston, Massachusetts

HELENE ELTCHANINOFF, MD
Professor of Medicine, Head of Department,
Department of Cardiology, Charles Nicolle
University Hospital, Rouen, France

TED FELDMAN, MD, FESC, FACC, FSCAI
Director, Cardiac Catheterization Laboratory,
NorthShore University HealthSystem,
Evanston, Illinois

EBERHARD GRUBE, MD
Medizinische Klinik und Poliklinik II,
Universitätsklinikum Bonn, Rheinische
Friedrich-Wilhelms-Universität, Bonn,
Germany

ZIYAD M. HIJAZI, MD, MPH
James A. Hunter University Chair, Professor of
Pediatrics and Internal Medicine; Director,
Section Chief, Pediatric Cardiology, Rush
Center for Congenital & Structural Heart
Disease, Rush University Medical Center,
Chicago, Illinois

IGNACIO INGLESSIS-AZUAJE, MD
Director, Adult Congenital Heart Disease
Intervention, Assistant Professor of Medicine,
Division of Cardiology, Massachusetts General
Hospital and Harvard Medical School, Boston,
Massachusetts

DAMIEN KENNY, MD
Rush Center for Congenital and Structural
Heart Disease, Rush University Medical
Center, Chicago, Illinois

ANNAPOORNA S. KINI, MD
Associate Director of the Cardiac
Catheterization Laboratory; Associate
Professor of Medicine, Mount Sinai Medical
Center, New York, New York

CHAD KLIGER, MD
Structural and Congenital Heart Disease
Fellow, Lenox Hill Heart and Vascular Institute,
New York, New York

RODRIGO M. LAGO, MD
Interventional Cardiology and Structural Heart
Disease, Massachusetts General Hospital,
Harvard Medical School, Boston,
Massachusetts

RONAN MARGEY, MD, MRCPI
Fellow, Structural Heart Disease and
Interventional Cardiology, Division of
Cardiology, Massachusetts General Hospital
and Harvard Medical School, Boston,
Massachusetts

PEDRO R. MORENO, MD
Director of Translational Research, Cardiac
Catheterization Laboratory; Professor of
Medicine, Mount Sinai Medical Center,
New York, New York

RAJEEV L. NARAYAN, MD
Cardiovascular Diseases, Mount Sinai School
of Medicine, New York, New York

GEORG NICKENIG, MD
Medizinische Klinik und Poliklinik II,
Universitätsklinikum Bonn, Rheinische
Friedrich-Wilhelms-Universität, Bonn,
Germany

IGOR F. PALACIOS, MD, FSCAI
Director of Interventional Cardiology,
Cardiology Division, Heart Center,
Massachusetts General Hospital; Associate
Professor of Medicine, Harvard Medical
School, Boston, Massachusetts

ALICE PERLOWSKI, MD
NorthShore University HealthSystem,
Evanston, Illinois

**CARLOS E. RUIZ, MD, PhD, FACC,
FSCAI, FACP**
Professor of Pediatrics and Medicine, Director
of Structural and Congenital Heart Disease,
Lenox Hill Heart and Vascular Institute,
New York, New York

SAMIN K. SHARMA, MD, FSCAI, FACC
Director of Clinical Cardiology; Director
of Cardiac Catheterization Laboratory,
Mount Sinai Medical Center, New York,
New York

JAN-MALTE SINNING, MD
Medizinische Klinik und Poliklinik II,
Universitätsklinikum Bonn, Rheinische
Friedrich-Wilhelms-Universität, Bonn,
Germany

NIKOS WERNER, MD
Medizinische Klinik und Poliklinik II,
Universitätsklinikum Bonn, Rheinische
Friedrich-Wilhelms-Universität, Bonn,
Germany

Contents

> Calcific aortic stenosis (AS) is a common expression of aortic valve disease and increases in prevalence with advancing age. Recent studies have shown that calcific deposition in aortic valve leaflets is an actively regulated process with many pathophysiologic similarities to atherosclerosis. Surgical valve replacement is the definitive treatment of calcific AS, but many patients do not undergo surgery because of prohibitive comorbidities or other high-risk features. Balloon aortic valvuloplasty remains an option for temporary palliation and symptomatic relief, and continues to serve as a bridge to aortic valve replacement in certain patients with AS requiring temporary hemodynamic stabilization.

> Transcatheter aortic valve implantation (TAVI) with the Edwards SAPIEN valve has been shown to be highly beneficial to patients at high risk or with contraindications to surgical aortic valve replacement. The availability of both transfemoral and transapical approaches allows the technique to be applied in most patients. Optimal screening and technical proficiency are crucial for a successful and safe procedure. The technique poses many technical challenges in sick and fragile elderly patients. Thus, TAVI should remain confined to formally trained and proctored experienced physicians, in centers of expertise offering an optimal multidisciplinary collaboration.

> The field of transcatheter aortic valve implantation has been rapidly evolving. The Medtronic CoreValve first emerged on the landscape in 2004 with initial first human studies, and it is currently being studied in the Pivotal US trial. This article details the current experience with the self-expanding aortic valve with a focus on clinical results and ongoing challenges.

> Transcatheter aortic valve implantation (TAVI) is an alternative to surgical aortic valve replacement in high-risk patients with symptomatic severe aortic stenosis. Several upcoming devices will optimize and facilitate the procedure: periprosthetic aortic regurgitation will be reduced by larger prosthesis sizes and repositionable next-generation transcatheter heart valves. Alternative access routes and smaller sheaths will reduce the rate of vascular complications. Cerebral protection devices might reduce the rate of strokes and silent cerebral embolism. Abandonment of balloon valvuloplasty and rapid ventricular pacing might facilitate the procedure and improve

outcome. Thus, younger and healthier patients could benefit from TAVI in the near future.

Percutaneous Mitral Balloon Valvuloplasty for Patients with Rheumatic Mitral Stenosis

Igor F. Palacios and Dabit Arzamendi

Percutaneous balloon dilatation of stenotic cardiac valves is used for the treatment of pulmonic, mitral, aortic, and tricuspid stenosis. Percutaneous mitral balloon valvuloplasty (PMV) has been used successfully as an alternative to open or closed surgical mitral commissurotomy in the treatment of symptomatic rheumatic mitral stenosis. PMV produces good immediate hemodynamic outcome, low complication rates, and clinical improvement in the majority of patients. PMV is safe and effective and provides clinical and hemodynamic improvement in rheumatic mitral stenosis. PMV is the preferred form of therapy for relief of mitral stenosis for a selected group of patients with symptomatic mitral stenosis.

Percutaneous Treatment of Mitral Regurgitation: The MitraClip Experience

Alice Perlowski and Ted Feldman

The MitraClip device is a percutaneous catheter-delivered, implantable clip that reduces mitral regurgitation by approximating the edges of the mitral leaflets, creating an "edge-to-edge" repair. The MitraClip is the first percutaneous technology developed to provide a minimally invasive option for patients at high risk for traditional mitral valve surgery. Although percutaneous repair was less effective at reducing mitral regurgitation than conventional surgery in the EVEREST randomized trial, the procedure was associated with superior safety and similar improvements in clinical outcomes. Older, high-risk or inoperable patients with functional or degenerative mitral regurgitation seem to benefit most from this therapy.

Percutaneous Treatment of Primary and Secondary Mitral Regurgitation: Overall Scope of the Problem

Chad Kliger and Carlos E. Ruiz

Mitral regurgitation is a heterogeneous disorder requiring the understanding of complex mitral anatomy and pathophysiology. Advanced imaging has furthered our knowledge and ability to treat patients with this disorder. As the demand for less invasive treatment increases, a multitude of percutaneous options have emerged. This review is written for interventionalists to fully appreciate the overall scope of the problem of mitral regurgitation. Understanding and integrating mitral anatomy with pathophysiology, multimodality imaging, and current transcatheter mitral therapies are paramount for treating this disorder.

Percutaneous Techniques for the Treatment of Patients with Functional Mitral Valve Regurgitation

Rodrigo M. Lago, Roberto J. Cubeddu, and Igor F. Palacios

Percutaneous approaches to mitral regurgitation remain largely investigational. In the last decade, novel percutaneous strategies have opened new options in the treatment of valvular heart disease. Several studies are currently underway to determine the benefits of transcatheter mitral valve repair therapy. Transcatheter chordal procedures are being developed, including chordal cutting and chordal implantation. Transcatheter valve implantation in the mitral position might offer a desirable alternative in selected patients and has been accomplished in a compassionate fashion on rare occasions in patients who are not candidates for surgical valve repair or replacement.

Transcatheter balloon pulmonary valvuloplasty (BPV) is the standard of care in managing symptomatic patients with moderate-to-severe pulmonary valvular stenosis, or asymptomatic patients with severe pulmonary valvular stenosis or with moderate pulmonary stenosis and evidence of objective exercise intolerance or right ventricular dysfunction. This article discusses the incidence, causes, and pathophysiology of valvular pulmonary stenosis in adolescents and adults; its natural history and noninvasive evaluation; the current guideline-recommended indications for BPV; the technical aspects of performing BPV; the immediate and long-term outcomes after valvuloplasty; and the complications and safety of the procedure. Also discussed is the role of this procedure in neonatal critical pulmonary stenosis and in percutaneous pulmonary valve replacement for patients with prior pulmonic valve interventions or degenerated right ventricular pulmonary artery conduits.

In all cases of congenital valvar aortic stenosis (AS), reduced effective orifice area leads to obstruction to flow, usually resulting from thickening and reduced motion of the valve leaflets. The most severe cases of valvar AS present soon after birth, with low cardiac output secondary to left ventricular dysfunction. Interventional treatment options consist of open surgical valvotomy or balloon valvuloplasty, with both therapies providing excellent but usually only temporary relief of stenosis. This article focuses on balloon aortic valvuloplasty as a therapy for congenital valvar AS in infants and children, focusing on established techniques, outcomes, and future challenges.

Initial enthusiasm for balloon aortic valvuloplasty (BAV) as an alternative to surgical aortic valve replacement waned because of the perceived failure of the procedure to alter the natural history of calcific severe aortic valve stenosis (AS) and significant initial procedural morbidity. Despite technical and procedural advances, BAV has been reserved as a palliative procedure for patients who cannot undergo valve replacement or as a bridge to surgery in hemodynamically unstable patients. This article reviews the indications, technical aspects, and outcomes of BAV for calcific AS and discusses the current role of BAV in the era of transcatheter aortic valve replacement.

The development of transcatheter valvular therapeutics has revolutionized interventional cardiology over the past decade. Nonetheless, despite these prominent advances in percutaneous valve technology, numerous obstacles regarding safety and efficacy must be overcome before the precise clinical role of these devices becomes clear. This article discusses the current status of transcatheter valve replacement and repair as it pertains to the aortic and mitral valve and deliberates on the bright future of a promising tool that will drastically affect clinical interventional practice.

Interventional Cardiology Clinics

READ THE CLINICS ONLINE!
Access your subscription at:
www.theclinics.com

Foreword

A New Review Periodical, *Interventional Cardiology Clinics*

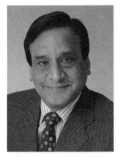 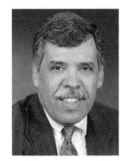

Samin K. Sharma, MD   Igor F. Palacios, MD
Consulting Editors

We are proud to share with you the introduction of a new review periodical, *Interventional Cardiology Clinics*. Beginning with this January 2012 issue, *Interventional Cardiology Clinics* will be published four times a year, in January, April, July, and October. Each issue will review a key topic in the field of interventional cardiology. *Interventional Cardiology Clinics* is a timely resource that fills the need for authoritative reviews to help physicians keep abreast with the rapidly developing trends in interventional cardiology. The topics that will be covered in 2012 include Coronary Interventions in Women, Chronic Total Occlusions, and STEMI Intervention.

This inaugural issue of *Interventional Cardiology Clinics* focuses on the field of structural heart disease. It comprises 12 selected topics written by experts in their field, who have provided succinct reviews that capture the most significant new information in this rapidly advancing area. We begin with an update on "Calcific Aortic Stenosis: Pathology and the Role of Balloon Aortic Valvuloplasty," followed by several articles on transcatheter aortic valve implantation, a procedure that has revolutionized the way we treat patients with severe aortic stenosis who are high surgical risk.

These articles include an overview of upcoming new devices and in-depth looks at the CoreValve and the Edwards SAPIEN device. Also highlighted are the expanded role of balloon aortic valvuloplasty in newborns and children, and its emergence in the era of transcatheter aortic valve implantation.

Special focus and attention are placed on the technical details of percutaneous treatment of mitral regurgitation, which are addressed in several articles. One article focuses on the MitraClip experience; others cover percutaneous mitral balloon valvuloplasty for patients with rheumatic mitral stenosis, percutaneous treatment of primary and secondary mitral regurgitation, and percutaneous techniques for the treatment of patients with functional mitral valve regurgitation. Most of these articles highlight a few recent randomized trials (Everest trials). All of them are presented in depth. Also included in the issue is an article on percutaneous therapies for pulmonary valvular stenosis.

Last, looking to the future of percutaneous treatment of patients with valvular heart disease is elaborated. Some of the articles have video components that may be viewed in the online version of this issue, which is available at

Intervent Cardiol Clin 1 (2012) xi–xii
doi:10.1016/j.iccl.2012.01.001

interventional.theclinics.com

http://www.interventional.theclinics.com/. We intend to make inclusion of videos a regular feature of *Interventional Cardiology Clinics*, since the visual aspect is vital to the field of interventional cardiology.

We are thankful to all the authors whose contributions have made this issue of *Interventional Cardiology Clinics* a valuable resource for interventional and clinical cardiologists and a future reference manual for technical details. The rapid advancements in the percutaneous treatment of structural heart disease are extending Andreas Gruentzig's dream of performing catheter-based percutaneous interventions with safety for all vascular (and valvular) disease states in alert, awake patients.

Samin K. Sharma, MD
Mount Sinai Heart
Box 1030, One Gustave L. Levy Place
New York, NY 10029-6754, USA

Igor F. Palacios, MD
Interventional Cardiology
Massachusetts General Hospital
55 Fruit Street, GRB 8, Suite 800
Boston, MA 02114, USA

E-mail addresses:
samin.sharma@mountsinai.org (S.K. Sharma)
ipalacios@partners.org (I.F. Palacios)

Calcific Aortic Stenosis: Pathology and Role of Balloon Aortic Valvuloplasty

Usman Baber, MD, MS, Annapoorna S. Kini, MD,
Pedro R. Moreno, MD, Samin K. Sharma, MD*

KEYWORDS

- Aortic stenosis • Balloon aortic valvuloplasty
- Aortic valve replacement

Aortic valve disease is a common manifestation of cardiac pathology, and calcific aortic stenosis (AS) is the leading indication for surgical aortic valve replacement (AVR) in the United States.[1] Characterized by a long latency period, symptom onset in calcific AS is associated with markedly reduced survival.[2] Three-year survival rates among symptomatic patients with severe AS who do not undergo AVR may be as low as 25%.[3] With the aging of the population, the overall burden and economic impact of AS is expected to increase as disease prevalence increases with age, affecting up to 4% of adults more than 85 years of age.[4,5] Although surgical AVR remains the definitive treatment of calcific AS,[6] many patients do not realize the benefits of this option because of extensive morbidity or other high-risk clinical and/or anatomic features.[7,8] Although not an alternative to AVR, balloon aortic valvuloplasty (BAV) provides temporary symptomatic and hemodynamic benefit in select patients with advanced AS. This article provides an overview of calcific AS disorders and assesses the role of BAV in the contemporary treatment of this disease entity.

SYMPTOMS OF AS

Multiple studies in the last 20 years suggest mechanistic similarities between AS and atherosclerosis. Population-based and epidemiologic studies have shown substantial overlap in risk factors for both diseases.[5,9,10] Data from the Cardiovascular Health Study found that older age, male gender, and hypertension were associated with aortic sclerosis.[9] Other studies have identified significant correlations between increased low-density lipoprotein (LDL) level, smoking, diabetes mellitus, and AS.[10]

In addition to these clinical associations, there are also similarities in the histopathologic features and clinical manifestations between atherosclerosis and AS. In a landmark pathologic study, Otto and colleagues[11] found that early AS lesions resemble those of atherosclerosis and are characterized by basement membrane disruption, lipid deposition, and a mononuclear cellular infiltrate comprising T cells and macrophages (**Fig. 1**). This shared pathologic substrate translates into a gradual and progressive clinical course across a continuum of disease severity in both AS and atherosclerosis. For example, morphologic changes to the aortic valve leaflets in the initial stages of AS do not result in left ventricular outflow obstruction precluding symptom onset. However, in a subset of patients with aortic sclerosis, there is progressive leaflet thickening, commissural fusion, and calcific deposition resulting in the cardinal AS symptoms of angina, syncope, and congestive heart failure.[2]

Despite the many similarities in histopathology and clinical factors between atherosclerosis and AS, the association is not necessarily causal and

Cardiac Catheterization Laboratory, Mount Sinai Medical Center, One Gustave L. Levy Place, Box 1030, New York, NY 10029, USA
* Corresponding author.
E-mail address: samin.sharma@mountsinai.org

Intervent Cardiol Clin 1 (2012) 1–9
doi:10.1016/j.iccl.2011.09.001
2211-7458/12/$ - see front matter Published by Elsevier Inc

interventional.theclinics.com

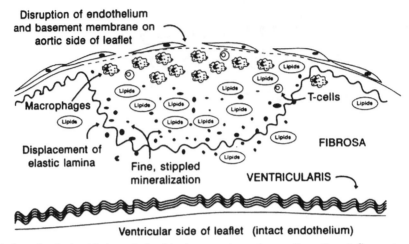

Disruption of endothelium and basement membrane on aortic side of leaflet

Macrophages

Lipids

T-cells

FIBROSA

Displacement of elastic lamina

Fine, stippled mineralization

VENTRICULARIS

Ventricular side of leaflet (intact endothelium)

Fig. 1. Early lesion of valvular AS characterized by basement membrane disruption, inflammatory cellular infiltrate, and lipid deposition. (*From* Otto CM, Kuusisto J, Reichenbach DD, et al. Characterization of the early lesion of 'degenerative' valvular aortic stenosis. Histologic and immunohistochemical studies. Circulation 1994;90(2): 851; with permission.)

important differences exist between the 2 conditions. For example, calcification tends to occur earlier and is a more prominent feature of AS compared with atherosclerosis. In addition, although smooth muscle cells are prominent in atherosclerosis, fibroblasts and myofibroblasts are the dominant cell types in AS.

Studies in the last 20 years have shown that endothelial dysfunction, lipid deposition, and chronic inflammation are critical pathologic features of AS. Other important pathologic features are shown in **Box 1**.

Endothelial Dysfunction

Endothelial cells lining the vascular tree are critical regulators of cellular and hemostatic integrity. Disruption of this cellular layer, or endothelial dysfunction, is a necessary initial step in the pathogenesis of both atherosclerosis and AS.[12–14] Moreover, the unique vulnerability of endothelial cells to areas of high mechanical and low shear stress

provides mechanistic insight into the regional variation of both atherosclerotic and AS lesions.[12] For example, atherosclerotic plaques tend to occur in branch points of the vasculature such as the infrarenal abdominal aorta and carotid bifurcation where mechanical stress is greatest but shear forces are low.[15,16] In a similar fashion, AS lesions localize on the aortic rather than the ventricular surface of the aortic valve because mechanical stress is highest in the flexion area near the aortic root attachment.[17] Moreover, a plausible rationale for why the noncoronary cusp is often the first cusp affected in AS is the absence of diastolic coronary flow leading to less shear stress across this cusp compared with the right and left coronary cusps.[17] Other lines of evidence also support a strong link between endothelial dysfunction and AS. Bicuspid aortic valves are subject to greater mechanical stress than their trileaflet counterparts, leading to earlier disease onset and symptoms.[18,19] In a clinical study, Poggianti and colleagues[20] also found that endothelium-dependent flow-mediated dilatation (FMD), a marker of systemic endothelial function, was significantly lower in patients with, versus without, aortic sclerosis (2.2% ± 3.5% vs 5.5 ± 5.5%, $P<.01$). Higher expression of endothelial markers including CD31, CD34, and von Willebrand factor in AS specimens compared with normal valves support greater activation of endothelial cells in AS disease progression.[21]

Lipid Deposition

Although investigators have documented the presence of lipid within stenotic aortic valves for more

---

Box 1
Important pathologic features of AS

Endothelial dysfunction

Lipid deposition

Chronic inflammation

Active regulated calcific phenotype in late-stage disease

Genetic polymorphisms that increase AS susceptibility

than 100 years, more recent clinical, histopathologic, and experimental studies have now begun to elucidate the sources and entry mechanisms of these lipoproteins and their subsequent impact on valvular calcification and inflammation. Several clinical studies have consistently shown positive associations between increases in plasma LDL and/or lipoprotein (a) with aortic valve sclerosis or stenosis.[22-24] In a separate report, Pohle and colleagues[25] examined the impact of plasma LDL on the extent and rate of progression of aortic valve calcification among patients with AS. The mean rate of progression of aortic valve calcification over 15 months was substantially higher in those with, versus without, increased LDL (9% $\pm$ 22% vs 43% $\pm$ 44%, $P<.001$). Moreover, LDL-C was linearly associated with annualized progression of aortic valve calcification ($r = 0.35$, $P<.001$). Histopathologic studies provide further insight and provide a biologic basis for these clinical observations. O'Brien and colleagues[22] were among the first to show that lipoproteins present in stenotic aortic valves contained the atherogenic apolipoproteins (apo) B, apo(a), and apo E. The presence of apo B within aortic valve lesions suggests not only that its source is circulating plasma LDL but also that its entry into the aortic valve may be partially mediated by extracellular matrix proteoglycans, analogous to lipoprotein uptake in atherosclerotic lesions.[26] Lipoproteins bind to proteoglycans via interactions between positively charged basic amino acids on apolipoproteins and negatively charged glycosaminoglycan side chains of proteoglycans.[26] In addition, other studies have colocalized specific apolipoproteins with particular proteoglycans.[27] In a surgical pathologic study, Olsson and colleagues[24] found that oxidized LDL (oxLDL) colocalized with areas of inflammation and calcification in stenotic aortic valve specimens. The clinical relevance of these findings is highlighted by oxidized cholesterol stimulating both calcified nodule formation by valve fibroblasts and inflammatory activity.[28] In aggregate, these studies provide a link between increased plasma LDL and lipoprotein (a) and increased AS risk.

Chronic Inflammation

Inflammation plays an important role in AS pathogenesis and disease progression. Several reports have documented that inflammatory cells including monocytes and T lymphocytes predominate in early AS lesions.[11,29,30] Monocytes differentiate into macrophages after entering the subendothelium. Other inflammatory cytokines and effector molecules have also been observed in stenotic aortic valves, including transforming growth factor-β1 (TGF-β1),[31] interleukin-1β,[32] tumor necrosis factor (TNF)-α,[33] and the terminal complement complex C5b-9.[34] These inflammatory mediators seem to exert their influence largely via regulation of additional enzymes and molecules involved in valvular remodeling and calcification. For example, the osteogenic cytokine TGF-β1 promotes calcification in aortic smooth muscle cells[35] and is a member of the same gene superfamily as the bone morphogenetic proteins.[36] Jian and colleagues[37] further evaluated the role of this cytokine in aortic valve calcification via immunohistochemistry and cell culture techniques and found higher levels of TGB-β1 in calcific human aortic valve cusps than in noncalcified cusps. The addition of TGB-β1 to sheep aortic valve interstitial cell culture led to apoptosis followed by calcification.[37] These provocative in vitro studies suggest a mechanistic pathway by which an inflammatory mediator, TGF-β1, might promote aortic valvular calcification via an apoptotic mechanism. Additional support for the important role of inflammation in the pathogenesis of AS was recently reported in a histopathologic study by Moreno and colleagues.[38] They found a significant increase in both inflammatory cellular infiltration and extent of calcification in bicuspid aortic valve specimens compared with trileaflet aortic valves.[38] Because congenital bicuspid AS is associated with more rapid progression and calcification, these findings provide further evidence for the important overlapping roles of inflammation and calcification in AS.

Calcification

The pathologic and clinical hallmark of advanced AS is extensive calcification, leading to leaflet rigidity and gradual left ventricular outflow obstruction. The higher prevalence of calcific AS in disease states associated with abnormal bone mineral metabolism, such as Paget disease and advanced chronic kidney disease, provides further evidence for the strong link between calcification and AS.[39,40] The adverse impact of valvular calcification in patients with AS was shown in a landmark report by Rosenhek and colleagues.[41] In this observational study of 128 patients with severe AS, the presence of aortic valve calcification was a robust discriminator of event-free survival because 2-year survival was significantly lower in patients with moderate to severe versus none or mild calcification (47% vs 84%, $P<.001$, **Fig. 2**).[41]

Although the presence of calcification in stenotic aortic valves is not a novel finding, recent

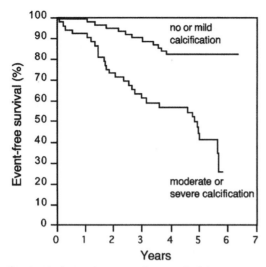

Fig. 2. Kaplan-Meier event-free survival for patients with asymptomatic AS with no or mild calcification compared with patients having moderate or severe aortic valve calcification. (*From* Rosenhek R, Klaar U, Schemper M, et al. Mild and moderate aortic stenosis. Natural history and risk stratification by echocardiography. Eur Heart J 2004;25(3):203; with permission.)

studies have established that calcific deposition does not occur passively but is an actively regulated process involving multiple cell types and pathways. Mohler and colleagues[28] found that human aortic valve cells in culture were able to differentiate into an osteoblast phenotype capable of mineralization. Moreover, the rate of calcified nodule formation by valvular interstitial cells was enhanced by TGF-β1 and bone morphogenetic protein 2.[28] Extending these observations, Rajamannan and colleagues[42] compared the genetic expression of various bone markers in calcific aortic valves with controls. Results of their ex vivo experiments showed significant upregulation in the diseased valves of genes encoding multiple osteogenic markers including osteocalcin, osteopontin, bone sialoprotein, and the osteoblast-specific transcription factor Cbfa1.[42] Multiple molecular pathways that are the subject of ongoing and intense investigation are involved in the complex regulation of pathologic calcification in advanced AS.[43–45]

TREATMENT OF AS

Surgical aortic valve replacement remains the preferred and definitive treatment of severe calcific AS with a class I indication in the most recent American College of Cardiology/American Heart Association valvular guidelines.[46] Relief of left ventricular outflow obstruction via surgical AVR results in regression of left ventricular hypertrophy, improvement in left ventricular function, and sustained symptomatic benefit.[47–49] In the absence of definitive therapy, severe AS is associated with significantly reduced survival, as shown in a retrospective study by O'Keefe and colleagues.[3] In this report, 1-year, 2-year, and 3-year survival rates in patients with untreated severe AS were 57%, 37%, and 25%, respectively.[3] In contrast, the analogous survival rates in age-matched and sex-matched controls were 93%, 85%, and 77%, respectively. Despite the unambiguous benefits of surgical AVR, many patients are denied surgery either because of high-risk features or patient/physician refusal.[7,50] This was shown in the Euro Heart Survey, because approximately 32% of patients with severe valvular heart disease did not undergo surgical treatment.[50] BAV, which involves increasing the aortic valve orifice via balloon dilatation, is a nonsurgical option for patients with severe AS who may be unable or unwilling to undergo surgery.

BAV: Technical Approaches and Complications

First introduced by Cribier and colleagues[51] in 1986 as a nonsurgical alternative to AVR, percutaneous BAV remains an important therapeutic option for thousands of patients with severe calcific AS who either refuse or are precluded from surgery because of multiple comorbidities. BAV may be performed either using a retrograde (brachial or femoral artery) or anterograde (transseptal) approach.

Although more commonly used and less technically demanding, the retrograde approach requires vascular anatomy suitable for large-caliber sheaths, which is a particularly relevant concern in the elderly AS population with multiple comorbid conditions that often include peripheral arterial disease. In addition, bleeding complications are greater because of the requirement of an arterial rather than venous access. In contrast, the technical challenges of anterograde BAV include transseptal puncture and balloon delivery across the left ventricular apex. Another potential complication of this approach is the creation of an atrial septal defect in up to 5% of patients, resulting in left-to-right shunts.[52] This small increase in cardiac output might result in an erroneous and falsely increased valve area calculation after anterograde BAV.[52]

Although there are no randomized comparisons of the 2 approaches, observational data suggest similar hemodynamic and clinical results with either technique.[53,54] In the largest series to date,

Cubeddu and colleagues[54] conducted a single-center, retrospective analysis of 157 patients with AS who underwent either anterograde (n = 46) or retrograde (n = 111) BAV. Although most baseline characteristics were well balanced in the 2 groups, the frequency of peripheral arterial disease was significantly higher in those undergoing anterograde BAV (41% vs 18%, P<.01). There were no differences in hemodynamic parameters including mean change in aortic valve area or peak gradient after BAV in the 2 groups. Despite a higher rate of vascular complications with the retrograde technique, there were no differences in clinical outcomes at 2 years.

Periprocedural complications are common during BAV and reflect both technical complexity and a high-risk patient mix. These complications include, but are not limited to, death, ischemic stroke, bleeding, and acute aortic regurgitation. Rates of transfusion, cerebrovascular accident, and mortality in the National Heart, Lung and Blood Institute (NHLBI) balloon valvuloplasty registry were 23%, 3%, and 3%, respectively.[55] Although technical improvements and better patient selection have led to a modest reduction in complication rates in the last 20 years,[56] periprocedural morbidity remains high. Balancing immediate procedural risk with any potential symptomatic improvement is therefore a critical component in the evaluation of any patient undergoing BAV.

BAV: Early Hemodynamic and Clinical Impact

Most studies have documented modest but significant improvements in various hemodynamic parameters including transaortic gradient, cardiac output, and aortic valve area (AVA) after BAV.[55–60] Although results vary according to severity of underlying AS and technique, reductions in peak gradient range between 30% and 40% with similar improvements in AVA. In the NHLBI registry, BAV was associated with a significant reduction in peak aortic gradient from 65 mm Hg to 31 mm Hg (P<.001) and a concordant increase in AVA from 0.5 cm^2 to 0.8 cm^2 (P<.001).[55] Similarly, Agarwal and colleagues[58] reported a significant reduction in peak transaortic gradient from 55 (± 22) to 20 (± 11) mm Hg and an increase in AVA from 0.6 (± 0.2) to 1.2 (± 0.3) cm^2 in a series of 212 patients with severe AS undergoing BAV. Immediate symptomatic improvement is also common after BAV and is consistent with the favorable changes in postprocedure hemodynamics. In general, this is reflected as reductions in New York Heart Association (NYHA) functional class. Data from the NHLBI demonstrated that 75% of patients surviving BAV at 30 days improved by at least 1 NYHA functional class or were unchanged if already class I at baseline.[55]

BAV: Long-term Results and Predictors of Survival

Despite early improvements in clinical and hemodynamic parameters, benefits are not sustained because midterm and long-term outcomes after BAV remain poor.[55,60] This is attributable both to high rates of restenosis and extensive morbidity in the AS population. Serial echocardiographic and clinical assessments of patients after BAV indicate restenosis rates approaching 60% at 6 months. Among 28 patients who underwent BAV with subsequent echocardiographic follow-up at 3 months, Safian and colleagues[60] reported that the frequency of aortic valve restenosis was 43%. In a larger series, Otto and colleagues[61] compared echocardiographic findings in 187 patients before and 6 months after BAV. Despite an immediate increase in AVA from 0.57 cm^2 to 0.78 cm^2 after BAV, mean AVA at 6 months was reduced to 0.65 cm^2.

Consistent with the high frequency of restenosis, survival after BAV is also poor.[56,59] Agarwal and colleagues[58] reported 1-year, 3-year, and 5-year survival rates after BAV of 64%, 28%, and 14%, respectively (**Fig. 3**). These rates are slightly higher than the 1-year and 3-year survival rates of 55% and 23% reported by Otto and colleagues.[61] Differences in survival rates after BAV in these 2 studies might be attributable to the impact of repeat BAV on long-term outcome. In the report by Agarwal and colleagues,[58] 24% of patients underwent an additional BAV, which emerged as an independent correlate of lower mortality (HR 0.88, 95% CI 0.80–0.95, P = .02).[58] However, such poor outcomes are not uniform in all patients after BAV and further risk stratification to identify patients who might realize a greater and sustained benefit is possible. Most studies have found that correlates of long-term survival after BAV are not related to procedural variables but reflect baseline morbidity and left ventricular performance. Agarwal and colleagues[58] found that independent predictors of mortality in patients surviving BAV included female gender, chronic renal insufficiency, the Charlson comorbidity index, and multiple BAV procedures. Similarly, Otto and colleagues[61] reported the following clinical, echocardiographic, and catheterization predictors of survival: functional status, left ventricular systolic function, cardiac output, cachexia, renal function, mitral regurgitation, and female gender. Several studies with sufficiently large sample sizes have identified strong discriminators of long-term risk

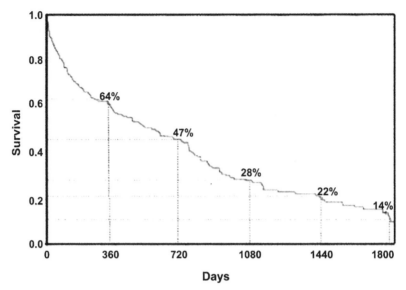

Fig. 3. Kaplan-Meier cumulative survival curves in 212 patients with severe AS who underwent BAV. (*From* Agarwal A, Kini AS, Attanti S, et al. Results of repeat balloon valvuloplasty for treatment of aortic stenosis in patients aged 59–104 years. Am J Cardiol 2005;95(1):46; with permission.)

after BAV. Klein and colleagues[56] found that the strongest predictor of mortality in 78 patients undergoing BAV was age and that each 10-year increment in age was associated with a twofold increase in mortality (RR 2.0, 95% CI 1.2–3.3, $P = .005$). There was a substantial difference in median survival in patients younger than, versus older than, 70 years of age (29.3 months vs 5.7 months, $P = .013$). After stratifying patients into low or high levels of risk using baseline assessments of left ventricular function and functional status, Otto and colleagues[61] compared long-term survival between groups. In the low-risk group, 1-year, 2-year, and 3-year survival rates were 76%, 53%, and 36%, respectively. The analogous rates in the high-risk group were 47%, 28%, and 17%. In aggregate, these data suggest that, although outcomes after BAV remain poor, improved patient selection might identify patients with more favorable and sustained benefit.

BAV in the Era of Transcatheter Aortic Valve Implantation

Transcatheter aortic valve implantation (TAVI) has emerged as a viable therapeutic alternative to surgical AVR. Initial single-center and multi-center experiences showed that this procedure is both safe and efficacious.[62,63] Among patients with severe AS at prohibitive surgical risk, results of The Placement of Aortic Transcatheter Valves (PARTNER) trial recently showed that TAVI is associated with marked reduction in mortality

compared with medical therapy alone.[64] In this landmark study, 358 patients with severe AS who were not suitable candidates for surgery were randomly allocated to standard therapy, including BAV, or transfemoral TAVI. BAV was performed in all patients before TAVI and in 84% of patients receiving standard therapy. All-cause mortality at 1 year was significantly reduced with TAVI (30.7% vs 50.7%, $P<.001$). With ongoing evolution of this technology and its active evaluation in lower-risk patients, the scope and applicability of TAVI is expected to increase. Although current guidelines endorse a limited and largely palliative role for the use of BAV,[46] the introduction of TAVI has spurred greater enthusiasm for this procedure.[57] In part, this reflects the need for a BAV in many patients before performing TAVI. AVR, either via surgical or transcatheter approaches, after BAV results in significantly improved survival compared with BAV alone. Lieberman and colleagues[59] reported 1-year survival of 52% in patients treated with BAV alone compared with 95% in those who underwent subsequent surgical AVR. Similar results were reported in a more contemporary series of patients who underwent either surgical AVR or TAVI after BAV.[57] These results indicate that BAV, either performed as an adjunctive or bridge procedure, remains relevant in the treatment of severe calcific AS.

SUMMARY

Pathophysiologic insights and treatment approaches to severe calcific AS have undergone substantial changes in the last 20 to 30 years. No longer considered an inevitable or degenerative process of aging, calcific deposition of the aortic valve is now understood to be an actively regulated process similar to atherosclerosis. In addition, TAVI offers a nonsurgical treatment alternative for selected patients with advanced AS. Within this contemporary framework, BAV will continue to play an important, albeit different, role in AS therapy. As Western populations continue to age, the incidence and prevalence of calcific AS will also increase. As such, treatment options for patients with advanced AS and extensive comorbidity or truncated life expectancy precluding TAVI will continue to be in demand. In such patients, BAV as a stand-alone procedure might provide palliative and significant symptom relief. Many patients with AS with hemodynamic instability or rapid clinical deterioration might also require BAV as a temporizing procedure before definitive surgical or transcatheter valve replacement. The important role of BAV as a bridge to AVR has been shown by several studies demonstrating a significant survival benefit compared with BAV alone. Ongoing studies will continue to enhance understanding of AS and further refine the role of BAV in the TAVI era.

REFERENCES

1. Lindroos M, Kupari M, Heikkila J, et al. Prevalence of aortic valve abnormalities in the elderly: an echocardiographic study of a random population sample. J Am Coll Cardiol 1993;21(5):1220–5.
2. Ross J Jr, Braunwald E. Aortic stenosis. Circulation 1968;38(Suppl 1):61–7.
3. O'Keefe JH Jr, Vlietstra RE, Bailey KR, et al. Natural history of candidates for balloon aortic valvuloplasty. Mayo Clin Proc 1987;62(11):986–91.
4. Nkomo VT, Gardin JM, Skelton TN, et al. Burden of valvular heart diseases: a population-based study. Lancet 2006;368(9540):1005–11.
5. Stewart BF, Siscovick D, Lind BK, et al. Clinical factors associated with calcific aortic valve disease. Cardiovascular Health Study. J Am Coll Cardiol 1997;29(3):630–4.
6. Bonow RO, Carabello BA, Chatterjee K, et al. 2008 Focused update incorporated into the ACC/AHA 2006 guidelines for the management of patients with valvular heart disease: a report of the American College of Cardiology/American Heart Association Task Force on Practice Guidelines (Writing Committee to Revise the 1998 Guidelines for the Management of Patients with Valvular Heart Disease). Endorsed by the Society of Cardiovascular Anesthesiologists, Society for Cardiovascular Angiography and Interventions, and Society of Thoracic Surgeons. J Am Coll Cardiol 2008;52(13):e1–142.
7. Bach DS, Siao D, Girard SE, et al. Evaluation of patients with severe symptomatic aortic stenosis who do not undergo aortic valve replacement: the potential role of subjectively overestimated operative risk. Circ Cardiovasc Qual Outcomes 2009;2(6):533–9.
8. Bouma BJ, van Den Brink RB, van Der Meulen JH, et al. To operate or not on elderly patients with aortic stenosis: the decision and its consequences. Heart 1999;82(2):143–8.
9. Mohler ER, Sheridan MJ, Nichols R, et al. Development and progression of aortic valve stenosis: atherosclerosis risk factors–a causal relationship? A clinical morphologic study. Clin Cardiol 1991;14(12):995–9.
10. Aronow WS, Ahn C, Kronzon I, et al. Association of coronary risk factors and use of statins with progression of mild valvular aortic stenosis in older persons. Am J Cardiol 2001;88(6):693–5.
11. Otto CM, Kuusisto J, Reichenbach DD, et al. Characterization of the early lesion of 'degenerative' valvular aortic stenosis. Histological and immunohistochemical studies. Circulation 1994;90(2):844–53.
12. Glagov S, Zarins C, Giddens DP, et al. Hemodynamics and atherosclerosis. Insights and perspectives gained from studies of human arteries. Arch Pathol Lab Med 1988;112(10):1018–31.
13. Yearwood TL, Misbach GA, Chandran KB. Experimental fluid dynamics of aortic stenosis in a model of the human aorta. Clin Phys Physiol Meas 1989;10(1):11–24.
14. Anderson TJ, Uehata A, Gerhard MD, et al. Close relation of endothelial function in the human coronary and peripheral circulations. J Am Coll Cardiol 1995;26(5):1235–41.
15. Zarins CK, Giddens DP, Bharadvaj BK, et al. Carotid bifurcation atherosclerosis. Quantitative correlation of plaque localization with flow velocity profiles and wall shear stress. Circ Res 1983;53(4):502–14.
16. Kjaernes M, Svindland A, Walloe L, et al. Localization of early atherosclerotic lesions in an arterial bifurcation in humans. Acta Pathol Microbiol Scand A 1981;89(1):35–40.
17. Freeman RV, Otto CM. Spectrum of calcific aortic valve disease: pathogenesis, disease progression, and treatment strategies. Circulation 2005;111(24):3316–26.
18. Beppu S, Suzuki S, Matsuda H, et al. Rapidity of progression of aortic stenosis in patients with congenital bicuspid aortic valves. Am J Cardiol 1993;71(4):322–7.
19. Pachulski RT, Chan KL. Progression of aortic valve dysfunction in 51 adult patients with congenital bicuspid aortic valve: assessment and follow up by Doppler echocardiography. Br Heart J 1993;69(3):237–40.
20. Poggianti E, Venneri L, Chubuchny V, et al. Aortic valve sclerosis is associated with systemic endothelial dysfunction. J Am Coll Cardiol 2003;41(1):136–41.

21. Chalajour F, Treede H, Ebrahimnejad A, et al. Angiogenic activation of valvular endothelial cells in aortic valve stenosis. Exp Cell Res 2004;298(2):455–64.

22. O'Brien KD, Reichenbach DD, Marcovina SM, et al. Apolipoproteins B, (a), and E accumulate in the morphologically early lesion of 'degenerative' valvular aortic stenosis. Arterioscler Thromb Vasc Biol 1996;16(4):523–32.

23. Walton KW, Williamson N, Johnson AG. The pathogenesis of atherosclerosis of the mitral and aortic valves. J Pathol 1970;101(3):205–20.

24. Olsson M, Thyberg J, Nilsson J. Presence of oxidized low density lipoprotein in nonrheumatic stenotic aortic valves. Arterioscler Thromb Vasc Biol 1999;19(5):1218–22.

25. Pohle K, Maffert R, Ropers D, et al. Progression of aortic valve calcification: association with coronary atherosclerosis and cardiovascular risk factors. Circulation 2001;104(16):1927–32.

26. Skalen K, Gustafsson M, Rydberg EK, et al. Subendothelial retention of atherogenic lipoproteins in early atherosclerosis. Nature 2002;417(6890):750–4.

27. O'Brien KD, Olin KL, Alpers CE, et al. Comparison of apolipoprotein and proteoglycan deposits in human coronary atherosclerotic plaques: colocalization of biglycan with apolipoproteins. Circulation 1998;98(6):519–27.

28. Mohler ER 3rd, Chawla MK, Chang AW, et al. Identification and characterization of calcifying valve cells from human and canine aortic valves. J Heart Valve Dis 1999;8(3):254–60.

29. Olsson M, Dalsgaard CJ, Haegerstrand A, et al. Accumulation of T lymphocytes and expression of interleukin-2 receptors in nonrheumatic stenotic aortic valves. J Am Coll Cardiol 1994;23(5):1162–70.

30. Olsson M, Rosenqvist M, Nilsson J. Expression of HLA-DR antigen and smooth muscle cell differentiation markers by valvular fibroblasts in degenerative aortic stenosis. J Am Coll Cardiol 1994;24(7):1664–71.

31. Anger T, Pohle FK, Kandler L, et al. VAP-1, Eotaxin3 and MIG as potential atherosclerotic triggers of severe calcified and stenotic human aortic valves: effects of statins. Exp Mol Pathol 2007;83(3):435–42.

32. Kaden JJ, Dempfle CE, Grobholz R, et al. Interleukin-1 beta promotes matrix metalloproteinase expression and cell proliferation in calcific aortic valve stenosis. Atherosclerosis 2003;170(2):205–11.

33. Kaden JJ, Dempfle CE, Grobholz R, et al. Inflammatory regulation of extracellular matrix remodeling in calcific aortic valve stenosis. Cardiovasc Pathol 2005;14(2):80–7.

34. Helske S, Oksjoki R, Lindstedt KA, et al. Complement system is activated in stenotic aortic valves. Atherosclerosis 2008;196(1):190–200.

35. Watson KE, Bostrom K, Ravindranath R, et al. TGF-beta 1 and 25-hydroxycholesterol stimulate osteoblast-like vascular cells to calcify. J Clin Invest 1994;93(5):2106–13.

36. Miyazono K, Kusanagi K, Inoue H. Divergence and convergence of TGF-beta/BMP signaling. J Cell Physiol 2001;187(3):265–76.

37. Jian B, Narula N, Li QY, et al. Progression of aortic valve stenosis: TGF-beta1 is present in calcified aortic valve cusps and promotes aortic valve interstitial cell calcification via apoptosis. Ann Thorac Surg 2003;75(2):457–65 [discussion: 465–6].

38. Moreno PR, Astudillo L, Elmariah S, et al. Increased macrophage infiltration and neovascularization in congenital bicuspid aortic valve stenosis. J Thorac Cardiovasc Surg 2011;142(4):895–901.

39. Maher ER, Pazianas M, Curtis JR. Calcific aortic stenosis: a complication of chronic uraemia. Nephron 1987;47(2):119–22.

40. Strickberger SA, Schulman SP, Hutchins GM. Association of Paget's disease of bone with calcific aortic valve disease. Am J Med 1987;82(5):953–6.

41. Rosenhek R, Klaar U, Schemper M, et al. Mild and moderate aortic stenosis. Natural history and risk stratification by echocardiography. Eur Heart J 2004;25(3):199–205.

42. Rajamannan NM, Subramaniam M, Rickard D, et al. Human aortic valve calcification is associated with an osteoblast phenotype. Circulation 2003;107(17):2181–4.

43. Caira FC, Stock SR, Gleason TG, et al. Human degenerative valve disease is associated with up-regulation of low-density lipoprotein receptor-related protein 5 receptor-mediated bone formation. J Am Coll Cardiol 2006;47(8):1707–12.

44. Kaden JJ, Bickelhaupt S, Grobholz R, et al. Receptor activator of nuclear factor kappaB ligand and osteoprotegerin regulate aortic valve calcification. J Mol Cell Cardiol 2004;36(1):57–66.

45. Steinmetz M, Skowasch D, Wernert N, et al. Differential profile of the OPG/RANKL/RANK-system in degenerative aortic native and bioprosthetic valves. J Heart Valve Dis 2008;17(2):187–93.

46. Bonow RO, Carabello BA, Chatterjee K, et al. 2008 Focused update incorporated into the ACC/AHA 2006 guidelines for the management of patients with valvular heart disease: a report of the American College of Cardiology/American Heart Association Task Force on Practice Guidelines (Writing Committee to Revise the 1998 Guidelines for the Management of Patients with Valvular Heart Disease): endorsed by the Society of Cardiovascular Anesthesiologists, Society for Cardiovascular Angiography and Interventions, and Society of Thoracic Surgeons. Circulation 2008;118(15):e523–661.

47. Croke RP, Pifarre R, Sullivan H, et al. Reversal of advanced left ventricular dysfunction following aortic valve replacement for aortic stenosis. Ann Thorac Surg 1977;24(1):38–43.

48. Kennedy JW, Doces J, Stewart DK. Left ventricular function before and following aortic valve replacement. Circulation 1977;56(6):944–50.

49. Pantely G, Morton M, Rahimtoola SH. Effects of successful, uncomplicated valve replacement on ventricular hypertrophy, volume, and performance in aortic stenosis and in aortic incompetence. J Thorac Cardiovasc Surg 1978;75(3):383–91.

50. Iung B, Baron G, Butchart EG, et al. A prospective survey of patients with valvular heart disease in Europe: the Euro Heart Survey on Valvular Heart Disease. Eur Heart J 2003;24(13):1231–43.

51. Cribier A, Savin T, Saoudi N, et al. Percutaneous transluminal aortic valvuloplasty using a balloon catheter. A new therapeutic option in aortic stenosis in the elderly. Arch Mal Coeur Vaiss 1986;79(12): 1678–86 [in French].

52. Feldman T. Transseptal antegrade access for aortic valvuloplasty. Catheter Cardiovasc Interv 2000; 50(4):492–4.

53. Block PC, Palacios IF. Comparison of hemodynamic results of anterograde versus retrograde percutaneous balloon aortic valvuloplasty. Am J Cardiol 1987;60(8):659–62.

54. Cubeddu RJ, Jneid H, Don CW, et al. Retrograde versus antegrade percutaneous aortic balloon valvuloplasty: immediate, short- and long-term outcome at 2 years. Catheter Cardiovasc Interv 2009;74(2):225–31.

55. Percutaneous balloon aortic valvuloplasty. Acute and 30-day follow-up results in 674 patients from the NHLBI Balloon Valvuloplasty Registry. Circulation 1991;84(6):2383–97.

56. Klein A, Lee K, Gera A, et al. Long-term mortality, cause of death, and temporal trends in complications after percutaneous aortic balloon valvuloplasty for calcific aortic stenosis. J Interv Cardiol 2006; 19(3):269–75.

57. Ben-Dor I, Pichard AD, Satler LF, et al. Complications and outcome of balloon aortic valvuloplasty in high-risk or inoperable patients. JACC Cardiovasc Interv 2010;3(11):1150–6.

58. Agarwal A, Kini AS, Attanti S, et al. Results of repeat balloon valvuloplasty for treatment of aortic stenosis in patients aged 59 to 104 years. Am J Cardiol 2005; 95(1):43–7.

59. Lieberman EB, Bashore TM, Hermiller JB, et al. Balloon aortic valvuloplasty in adults: failure of procedure to improve long-term survival. J Am Coll Cardiol 1995;26(6):1522–8.

60. Safian RD, Warren SE, Berman AD, et al. Improvement in symptoms and left ventricular performance after balloon aortic valvuloplasty in patients with aortic stenosis and depressed left ventricular ejection fraction. Circulation 1988;78(5 Pt 1):1181–91.

61. Otto CM, Mickel MC, Kennedy JW, et al. Three-year outcome after balloon aortic valvuloplasty. Insights into prognosis of valvular aortic stenosis. Circulation 1994;89(2):642–50.

62. Himbert D, Descoutures F, Al-Attar N, et al. Results of transfemoral or transapical aortic valve implantation following a uniform assessment in high-risk patients with aortic stenosis. J Am Coll Cardiol 2009;54(4):303–11.

63. Webb JG, Altwegg L, Boone RH, et al. Transcatheter aortic valve implantation: impact on clinical and valve-related outcomes. Circulation 2009;119(23): 3009–16.

64. Leon MB, Smith CR, Mack M, et al. Transcatheter aortic-valve implantation for aortic stenosis in patients who cannot undergo surgery. N Engl J Med 2010;363(17):1597–607.

Transcatheter Aortic Valve Implantation: Experience with the Edwards SAPIEN Device

Alain Cribier, MD*, Helene Eltchaninoff, MD

KEYWORDS

- Aortic stenosis • Transcatheter valve • Valve replacement
- Cardiac catheterization

It is recognized that about one-third of patients with symptomatic aortic stenosis (AS) are not offered surgical valve replacement.[1] Transcatheter aortic valve implantation (TAVI) was introduced in 2002[2] with the goal of offering an alternative treatment to patients with severe symptomatic AS who are poor candidates for conventional aortic valve replacement (AVR) because of their elevated mortality risk. The concept was validated by the authors' group in patients in whom implantation was done on a compassionate basis[3,4] with a first generation of balloon expandable valves (Percutaneous Valve Technologies, NJ, USA) and a transseptal venous approach. Since then, the devices and implantation techniques have considerably improved and TAVI has entered a common clinical reality. Two valve models, the balloon-expandable Edwards SAPIEN Valve (Edwards Lifescience, Irvine, CA, USA) and the self-expandable CoreValve Revalving System (CoreValve Inc, Irvine, CA, USA) are currently commercialized in Europe and have been used in more than 40,000 cases worldwide, and multiple other devices are under investigation.

Several feasibility trials and postmarket registries[5–13] have shown that using the Edwards SAPIEN prosthesis, TAVI can be performed safely and effectively using either the transfemoral retrograde or the transapical antegrade approaches with the potential for durable benefit. Recently, using the Edwards SAPIEN device, the prospective pivotal randomized Placement of Aortic Transcatheter Valve (PARTNER)-US trial has confirmed these findings.[14,15]

As a larger number of centers become involved in TAVI, careful patient selection and a meticulously performed procedure are required to maintain the outcomes published in clinical trials.

PRODUCT OVERVIEW
The Edwards SAPIEN Transcatheter Heart Valve

The Edwards SAPIEN Transcatheter Heart Valve (THV) consists of a tubular slotted stainless steel balloon expandable stent with an integrated unidirectional trileaflet bovine tissue valve with a polyethylene terephthalate fabric cuff (**Fig. 1**). The valve is made of 3 equal sections of bovine pericardium manufactured with the anticalcium ThermaFix treatment. The prosthesis is available in 2 sizes, with an expandable diameter of 23 or 26 mm and a length of 14 and 16 mm, respectively. The valve is compressed over the delivery balloon catheter using a crimping tool (**Fig. 2**) to symmetrically reduce its overall diameter from its expanded size to its mounted size (**Fig. 3**).

Disclosure: Alain Cribier is Consultant for Edwards Lifesciences. No other disclosure.
Department of Cardiology, Charles Nicolle University Hospital, 1 Rue de Germont, 76000 Rouen, France
* Corresponding author.
E-mail address: Alain.Cribier@chu-rouen.fr

Intervent Cardiol Clin 1 (2012) 11–25
doi:10.1016/j.iccl.2011.09.006

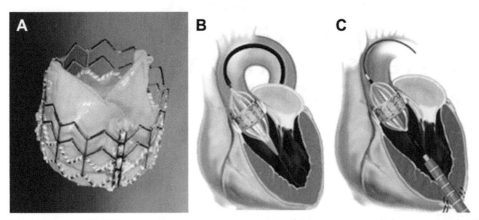

Fig. 1. (*A*) The Edwards-SAPIEN transcatheter heart valve consists of 3 bovine pericardial cusps treated with ThermaFix mounted into a stainless steel balloon expandable stent with a lower portion covered with polyethylene terephthalate cuff. Two approaches are used for THV implantation: (*B*) transfemoral and (*C*) transapical. (*Courtesy of* Edwards Lifesciences, Irvine, CA, USA; with permission.)

The Edwards SAPIEN THV can be delivered via a transfemoral or transapical approach (see **Fig. 1**) using the RetroFlex and Ascendra delivery systems (Edwards Lifesciences, Irvine, CA, USA), respectively.

The last generation of transfemoral delivery systems, the RetroFlex 3 (Edwards Lifesciences, Irvine, CA, USA) (see **Fig. 3**), consists of a deflectable balloon catheter with a distal nose cone that helps advancing the THV across vascular tortuosity, reducing the friction at the level of the aortic arch, crossing the native valve and increasing stability for accurate THV placement and delivery. Other components of the transfemoral kit are a 30 cm long hydrophilic-coated introducer sheath of 22F or 24F for the 23- and 26-mm THVs, respectively; polyethylene dilators of 16F to 28F for smooth arterial dilatation; and a RetroFlex balloon catheter of 20 or 23 mm in diameter, depending on the THV size, for predilatation of the native aortic valve (**Fig. 4**).

The transapical Ascendra delivery system (**Fig. 5**) allows a direct access to the native valve. The Ascendra introducer sheath is 26F in size and provides controlled insertion through the apex of the left ventricle. A 20-mm Ascendra balloon catheter is used for aortic valve predilatation.

PATIENT SELECTION
Clinical Criteria

Appropriate patient selection is crucial for a successful procedure. Clinical, anatomic, and functional characteristics affect procedural outcomes and have to be considered when evaluating potential candidates. TAVI should be restricted to patients with severe symptomatic AS who have a potential for functional improvement after the procedure, whereas using TAVI in patients with comorbidities affecting survival or quality of life remains questionable. In active elderly patients, TAVI adds important symptom relief and a survival advantage, but older

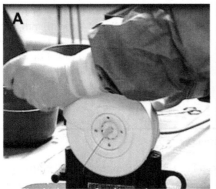
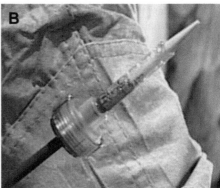

Fig. 2. (*A*) The crimping tool used for reducing the valve size to the mounted size. (*B*) After crimping, the valve is covered by a loader to facilitate its introduction within the arterial introducer.

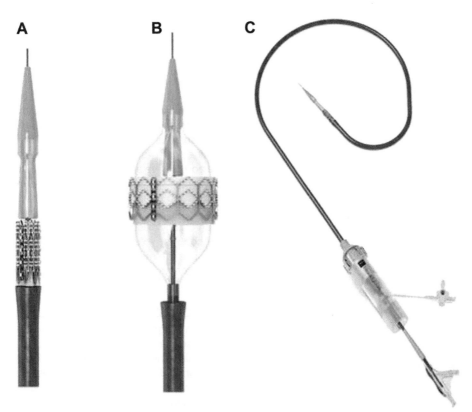

Fig. 3. (*A*) The valve is crimped at midpart of the balloon and (*B*) will be delivered by balloon inflation. (*C*) The Retroflex 3 delivery system. (*Courtesy of* Edwards Lifesciences, Irvine, CA, USA; with permission.)

patients receive a greater degree of functional improvement than a survival advantage compared with younger ones. Preoperative risk assessment is performed using the EuroSCORE or the Society of Thoracic Surgeons (STS) risk calculator for these patients.

In the absence of formal contraindication to surgical valve replacement, a EuroSCORE greater than 20% or an STS score greater than 10% is requested. However, a trend to include patients with lower risks (EuroScore >15%) is currently observed in Europe, whereas patient frailty,

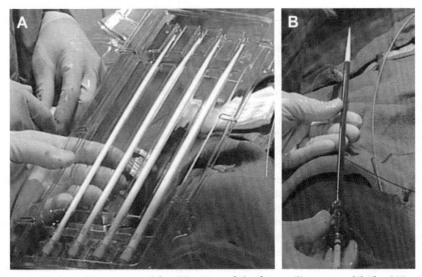

Fig. 4. (*A*) The polyethylene dilatators used for dilatation of the femoroiliac access. (*B*) The 24F arterial sheath.

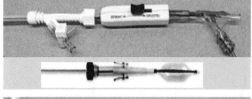

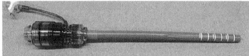

Fig. 5. The Ascendra delivery system used for the transapical approach. Proximal and distal ends of the delivery system (*upper panel*). The 26F sheath (*lower panel*). (*Courtesy of* Edwards Lifesciences, Irvine, CA, USA; with permission.)

whatever the score, has become another inclusion criteria. The indication of TAVI and the benefit/risk profile must be cautiously discussed for each patient by a multidisciplinary team (the heart team) of primary cardiologists, interventional cardiologists, cardiac surgeons, echocardiographers, radiologists, anesthesiologists, and geriatricians.

A stable condition before the procedure is required. Patients with decompensated heart failure and severely depressed left ventricular ejection fraction should undergo medical optimization and balloon aortic valvuloplasty (BAV) to allow improvement of their ventricular function as well as stress echocardiography to assess the myocardial contractility reserve. Patients with severe coronary artery disease with significant stenosis on main branches (left main, proximal left anterior descending, or right coronary artery) should undergo coronary angioplasty 2 to 3 weeks before TAVI.

Assessment of Arterial Access

Minimal luminal diameter, tortuosity, and calcification of the aorta, iliac and femoral arteries, must be closely assessed and influence the implantation route. Patients with small, heavily calcified, tortuous arteries should preferentially undergo TAVI through the transapical approach to prevent vascular complications. Minimal vessel diameters of 7 mm and 8 mm are required for sheath insertion in the transfemoral approach for the 22F and 24F sheaths, respectively, in the absence of calcification, but the diameter must be greater than the introducer size in case of circumferential arterial wall calcification, which increases the risk of dissection or rupture during sheath insertion or removal. Arterial characteristics must be evaluated by at least 2 different imaging modalities. Angiography is a simple method that gives a fairly good idea of vessel diameter and tortuosity. Contrast-enhanced computed tomographic angiography (CT Scan) is crucial and has the advantage of providing excellent vessel resolution noninvasively (**Fig. 6**). CT Scan evidences the severity of calcification and luminal diameter on cross section views and allows arterial 3-dimensional reconstruction. Noncontrasted CT Scan is an alternative in patients with chronic renal insufficiency. Thoracoabdominal CT Scan (**Fig. 7**) is also used in routine for a full assessment of the anatomy of the aortic valve and thoracic and abdominal aorta. However, because of the volume of contrast required to perform all preoperative tests (angiographies and CT Scan), a risk of contrast-induced nephropathy exists. Spacing the studies, decreasing the contrast volume, diluting the contrast media, and use of measures for nephroprotection are recommended.

Echocardiography

Echocardiography, either transthoracic (TTE) or transesophageal (TEE), plays a crucial role for assessing the severity of AS, the left ventricular function and wall thickness, the presence of associated valvular disease, and the diameter of the aortic annulus, which will determine the optimal THV size. This diameter is measured in the long-axis view at the level of the aortic leaflet insertion (**Fig. 8**). In the United States, The Edwards SAPIEN valves are compatible with annulus diameters of 18 to 24 mm. In Europe, a larger THV size (29 mm) is available for larger annulus diameters, its use being limited to the transapical approach. TTE provides accurate information in most patients, but TEE is useful in case of poor echogenicity. The diameter is generally found 1 mm smaller with TTE than with TEE, which is considered more exact. CT Scan can also be used to assess the aortic annulus dimension, even though the values are often 2 to 3 mm greater than with TTE and TEE. The prosthesis is sized according to the following values: a diameter of 18 to 21 mm requires a 23-mm valve, whereas a diameter greater than 21 mm requires a 26-mm valve. In questionable or borderline cases (diameter of 21 mm), optimal valve sizing remains uncertain before the procedure. In this setting, a 23-mm balloon should be systematically used for preimplantation valvotomy at the time of TAVI and aortogram performed during full balloon inflation. Assessment of the free space between balloon edges and aortic wall and the degree of paravalvular leak easily confirm the optimal bioprosthesis size.

Other factors that decrease procedural success or predict complications can be identified by echocardiography, angiography, CT Scan, and

A   B

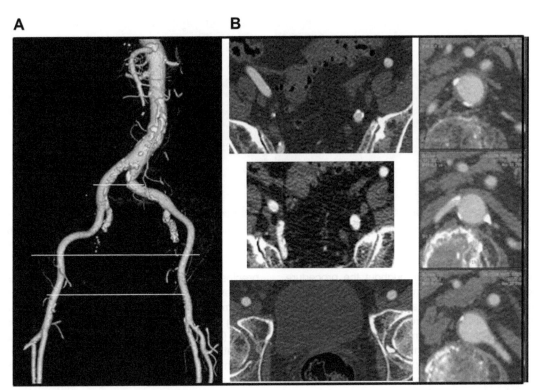

Fig. 6. Assessment of the femoroiliac access by CT Scan. (*A*) Three-dimensional reconstruction of the atrial access. (*B*) Cross-sectional views for qualitative (calcification) and quantitative (internal diameter) analysis of each arterial segment.

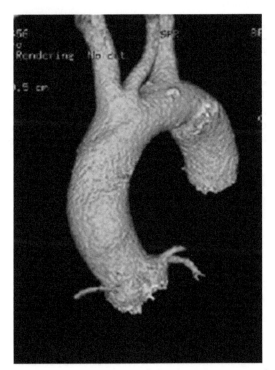

Fig. 7. CT Scan evaluation of the thoracic aorta used to detect its size, angulation, and calcification.

electrocardiography. Patients with bicuspid aortic valves are not optimal candidates for TAVI because the valvular orifice is elliptical and may predispose to perivalvular aortic insufficiency. Huge calcific valvular nodules can increase the risk of coronary occlusion after valve deployment and may contraindicate TAVI. A mitral prosthesis may also interfere with valve placement and is currently considered a relative contraindication to TAVI. A preexisting right bundle branch block may predispose to complete heart block and pacemaker dependency.[16]

The angulation between the ascending aorta and the heart influences the procedure as well. Horizontal aortic root with vertical aortic annulus may complicate valve positioning. Severe calcification of the aortic wall (porcelain aorta) in severely angulated aorta may increase the risk of aortic dissection and constitutes a better indication for the transapical approach.

TRANSFEMORAL PROCEDURE

Each procedural step is important and must be completed cautiously with constant observation of the patient's hemodynamic condition and permanent communication between operators and

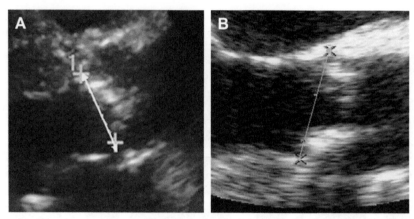

Fig. 8. The annulus diameter must be measured at the level of the leaflets insertion by TTE (*A*) or TEE (*B*) in the longitudinal view.

the paramedical team throughout the procedure. Adaptation of the conventional cardiac catheterization room to meet surgical sterility standards is very important. In this regard, surgical hybrid rooms would constitute an optimal setting.

Antiplatelet treatment includes aspirin and a loading dose of clopidogrel administered 24 hours before intervention and antibiotics (cephalosporin), given just before the procedure and continued for 48 hours thereafter. General anesthesia is optional for TAVI using the transfemoral approach. In the authors' institution, the procedure is performed under local anesthesia (lidocaine 2%) and sedation (midazolam, 2 mg intravenously [IV], and nalbuphine, 5 mg IV). Heparin, 50 U/kg IV is administered after cut down of the femoral artery at the groin. TEE should be rapidly available if necessary.

Arterial Access

Even though in experienced hands the transarterial access can be accomplished using a percutaneous preclose technique with percutaneous closure devices,[17] a surgical cut down is generally preferred, which allows direct control of the artery during sheath insertion and simplifies vascular repair (**Fig. 9**). The femoral artery with larger arterial diameter and less tortuosity is selected. Two sheaths are placed in the contralateral femoral artery and vein (6F and 7F, respectively) for placement of a pigtail catheter in the aorta and a pacemaker lead in the right ventricle. The anterior wall of the femoral artery is exposed, whereas the posterior wall is not dissected to facilitate sheath insertion.

Reference Aortogram

A supra-aortic angiogram is performed through the contralateral femoral artery to obtain a reference view of the aortic root and aortic annulus. The fluoroscopic projection is critical for appropriate valve placement because the line of valvular calcification is the landmark for valve positioning. In patients with poor calcification of the native

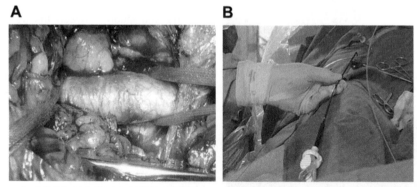

Fig. 9. (*A*) Aspect of the femoral artery after cut down at the groin. The less calcific zone is selected for cannulation. (*B*) In selected cases, a percutaneous approach can be performed. The technique requires the use of a preclosing device, here a Prostar (Abbott Inc, Chicago, IL, USA) 10F device.

valve, adjunct online TEE can be useful. The projection should show the aortic annular plane perpendicular to the screen, with the 3 aortic sinuses in line (**Fig. 10**). Generally, the incidence is anteroposterior or slightly left anterior oblique with cranial angulation. The reference view is displayed on a screen to facilitate balloon positioning at the time of valve predilatation and later on positioning of the prosthesis.

Test of Rapid Ventricular Pacing

Rapid ventricular pacing (RVP)-induced ventricular tachycardia accomplishes an optimal reduction of the cardiac output, creating a transient cardiac standstill. RVP, which was tried by the authors during BAV since 2001,[18] was successfully extended to TAVI[4,19] and seems to be crucial for accurate valve positioning. The pacing lead should be easily and reliably placed at the midpart of the right ventricle's posterior wall with low risk of dislodgement or ventricular perforation. The purpose of RVP is to pace at a rate that will bring the mean arterial pressure to less than 50 mm Hg. Generally this pressure is achieved at a heart rate of 200 or 220 beats per minute (BPM). If a 2:1 block occurs during stimulation, then the rate might be decreased to 180 BPM or the position of the lead modified. Lower pacing rates (160/150 BPM) are acceptable in case of severely depressed myocardial contractility. Optimal team coordination is required throughout the RVP procedure. All balloon inflations should start when the blood pressure reaches its nadir and the stimulation is stable (**Fig. 11**). The duration of pacing bursts should be as short as possible and the number of bursts minimized because it may cause significant hypotension and myocardial

depression, more particularly in patients with severe coronary artery disease and depressed ejection fraction.

Aortic Valve Predilatation

Dilating the native aortic valve is necessary to increase the effective orifice area and facilitates the placement of the stent/valve unit. The balloon catheter can be introduced through a 14F introducer or through the 22F or 24F sheath primarily placed within the exposed femoral artery. Crossing the native aortic valve is generally accomplished with an Amplatz Left 2 coronary catheter and a straight guidewire. Once the valve is crossed, a 260 cm long 0.035 in Amplatz Extra Stiff J Guidewire (COOK, Bjaeverskov, Denmark) is advanced within the left ventricle, which offers an optimal support for valve predilatation as for THV implantation. The distal floppy portion of the wire must be preshaped by hand in an exaggerated curve to limit the risk of left ventricular wall injury.

The balloon catheter used for BAV is the 40 mm long RetroFlex Valvotomy Catheter from Edwards Lifesciences (see **Fig. 8**). Two diameter sizes are available, 20 or 23 mm, depending on the THV size used (23 or 26 mm, respectively). The balloon, carefully purged of air, is advanced over the stiff wire and placed at midnative valve. A contrast dilution of 15:85 contrast media/saline solution is used for valvotomy. This dilution reduces viscosity, thus facilitating the inflation-deflation cycles. One or 2 inflations should be performed (**Fig. 12**). Subsequent inflations should not be performed until the patient's blood pressure normalizes. Simultaneous contrast injection and balloon inflation can be used to confirm aortic annulus size and evaluate coronary flow. Special

A   **B**

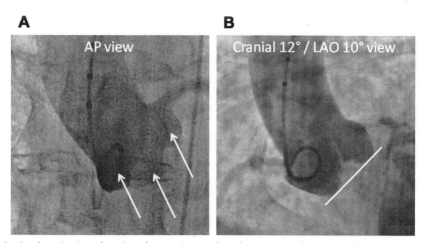

Fig. 10. (*A*) Optimal projection showing the aortic annular plane perpendicular to the screen with the 3 aortic sinuses (*arrows*) in line is crucial for accurate THV positioning. (*B*) In this example, alignment is obtained by changing the projection from anteroposterior to left anterior oblique 10°/cranial 12° angulation.

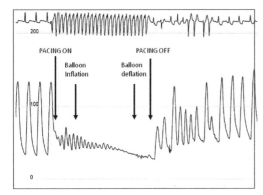

Fig. 11. Effect of a 5-second burst of rapid pacing on the aortic pressure. Start and discontinuation of pacing and balloon inflation/deflation are indicated by the arrows.

attention should be placed on the position of calcium nodules in relation to the coronary ostia because coronary occlusion has been reported after TAVI.[5]

Dilatation of the Arterial Access and Sheath Insertion

Progressive dilation of the femoral and iliac arteries must be performed in preparation to the large sheath insertion using polyethylene dilators of increasing size advanced over the wire. The 22F or 24F sheath is then cautiously inserted under visual control within the femoral artery and advanced into the descending aorta under fluoroscopic guidance (**Fig. 13**). In case of a significant resistance to progression, it is preferable to stop the procedure and change the intended placement route instead of experiencing a life-threatening vascular complication.

Valve Placement

The RetroFlex 3 is then introduced into the sheath and advanced to the aortic valve under fluoroscopic guidance (see **Fig. 13**). Crossing the aortic arch is performed in the left anterior oblique 40° view after flexion of the RetroFlex 3 aimed at decreasing the friction against the aorta's wall and the risk of plaque dislodgement. In the ascending aorta, the x-ray tube is moved to the reference projection and the RetroFlex 3 fully flexed, which allows, together with a slight back tension on the guidewire, crossing the native valve in its center. Before crossing the valve, a test of RVP must confirm optimal capture. The aortic valve is then crossed and the RetroFlex 3 withdrawn over the balloon catheter shaft by 3 to 4 cm to allow full balloon inflation without any interference while maintaining the bioprosthesis at the level of the native valve. Correct placement of the THV is the most critical step of the procedure and deserves significant attention. Before deployment, one-third to half of the stented prosthesis needs to rest above the annulus to minimize perivalvular leaks and avoid coronary occlusion. The valve plane seen as a strip of calcium in the fluoroscopy monitors is used as a landmark. In addition, contrast injections must be performed with a pigtail catheter advanced from the contralateral artery to the level of the valve plane.

Valve Deployment

Valve deployment (see **Fig. 13**) must be done under RVP. Balloon inflation is performed by manually injecting a 15:85 contrast/saline solution, the volume of which has been determined before valve crimping to obtain the optimal valve diameter (23 or 26 mm). RVP is started and the balloon

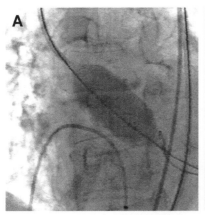
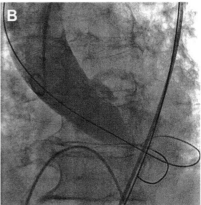

Fig. 12. (*A*) The 40 mm long, 23 mm in diameter RetroFlex Valvulotomy catheter is used for aortic valve predilatation, inflated across the aortic valve under rapid pacing. (*B*) A second inflation with aortogram is confirmed to validate the valve size and assess the potential risk of left main trunk occlusion.

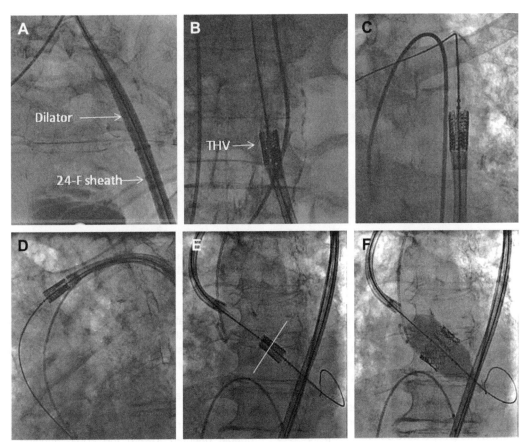

Fig. 13. (A) Insertion of the 24F RetroFlex (*arrow*) over its dilator (*arrow*) within the femoral artery. (B) The THV (*arrow*) is advanced within the sheath and (C) within the ascending aorta in the anteroposterior view. (D) The RetroFlex catheter is flexed to pass the aortic arch in the left anterior oblique 40° view and (E) advanced in the ascending aorta to cross the native valve in the reference view. THV positioning is obtained using the strip of calcium as a landmark (*white bar*). (F) The THV is deployed by balloon inflation under rapid pacing.

inflated after the blood pressure reaches its nadir and stabilizes. Full balloon inflation is maintained 3 to 5 seconds before deflation, and RVP can then be discontinued. The delivery catheter is then rapidly removed from the valve. Results are assessed by supra-aortic angiography (**Fig. 14**) and echocardiography.

Sheath Removal

The sheath must be removed as soon as the valve is deployed and its position corroborated. Sheath removal should be done after reinsertion of its dilator while maintaining the stiff guidewire in place in the descending aorta and with simultaneous contrast injection from the contralateral pigtail or a right internal mammary catheter placed at the level of iliac bifurcation. Covered stents and occlusion balloons should be available in the angiographic suite to treat arterial rupture. Flow-limiting dissections can be treated with noncovered stents, whereas complex arterial damage may require

emergent arterial reconstruction. Angiography should always be performed after vessel repair to confirm vessel patency and runoff.

Postimplantation Care

In case of general anesthesia, extubation should be attempted as soon as possible, in the catheterization room or soon after transfer in the intensive care unit. In the absence of complication, hospital discharge can be generally obtained 4 to 6 days after the procedure. In the absence of new left bundle branch block or atrioventricular block, the pacing lead can be removed immediately after the procedure. Older and very sick patients require special care, with close monitoring of hemodynamics and renal function.

TRANSAPICAL PROCEDURE

The transapical procedure is a minimally invasive off-pump surgical approach that should be ideally

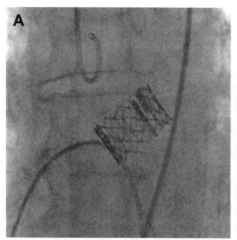 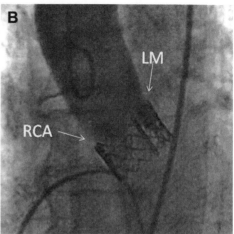

Fig. 14. (*A*) THV in place after delivery. (*B*) Supra-aortic angiography to assess the degree of aortic regurgitation and the patency of the coronary arteries. No aortic regurgitation and patency of the left main (LM) artery and right coronary artery (RCA) in this representative case.

performed in a hybrid operative theater offering optimal fixed fluoroscopy system as in conventional cardiac catheterization room, because the quality of imaging is a crucial factor for success. However, most of the procedures are currently performed in regular operative rooms, using high-quality mobile C-arm systems for imaging, or even in cardiac catheterization laboratories converted into an operative setting. The procedure is performed by a team of cardiac surgeons, interventional cardiologists, an anesthetist, and echocardiographers, under general anesthesia, with online TEE. Premedication is limited to aspirin (75 mg) and antibiotics. Clopidogrel is administered at patient's discharge. Heparin, 50 U/kg IV, is administered after cannulation of the left ventricle.

Reference Aortogram and RVP

Venous and femoral arterial sheaths are placed at the beginning of the procedure, and a pigtail catheter is advanced into the ascending aorta. The venous line can be used as an approach for the pacing lead even though epicardial pacing may be preferred in this setting. The reference view showing the aortic annular plane perpendicular to the screen is obtained by aortography. Test of RVP is obtained as for the transfemoral approach.

Operative Steps

Mini thoracotomy and purse-string suture
After detection of the left ventricular apex by TTE, anterolateral minithoracotomy is performed in the fifth or sixth intercostal space; the pericardium is open and the apex exposed (**Figs. 15** and **16**). The optimal puncture site is then determined, close

to the apex, lateral to the left anterior descending artery, and in the healthiest myocardial zone. Two apical purse-string sutures are performed using Prolene 2-0 thread, about 2 cm in diameter.

Crossing the aortic valve and valve predilatation
The ventricular puncture is then obtained, with the needle oriented toward the aortic annulus detected by fluoroscopy. A soft guidewire is then used for antegrade aortic valve crossing. TEE is required in case of any resistance to the progression of the wire within the left ventricle to detect incidental crossing of a mitral chorda. Through a 14F sheath introduced within the left ventricle and with the help of a right Judkins coronary catheter, the 260 cm long 0.035 in Amplatz Extra Stiff J Guidewire is positioned into the descending aorta. Balloon valvuloplasty can then be performed during a brief episode of RVP, using the Ascendra Valvotomy Catheter (Edwards Lifesciences, Irvine, CA, USA), which is 20 mm in diameter, irrespective of the THV size planned. After removal of the 14F sheath, the 26F transapical delivery catheter is inserted within the left ventricle, with the distal tip positioned 2 to 3 cm below the native aortic valve. The crimped THV connected to the sheath by its loader and correctly oriented can then be advanced over the stiff guidewire across the aortic valve.

Valve positioning and delivery
After removal of the pusher included within the delivery system, the THV is positioned as in the transfemoral approach, one-half or two-thirds below the aortic annulus detected by fluoroscopy

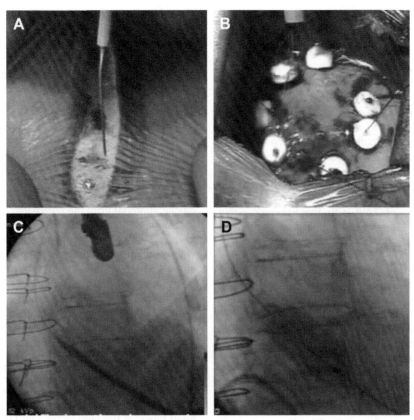

Fig. 15. Initial phases of the transapical approach: (*A*) minithoracotomy, (*B*) double apical purse-string suture, (*C*) native valve crossed with the 14F sheath, (*D*) balloon dilatation with the 20-mm Ascendra balloon catheter.

and TEE, with the help of repeated aortograms obtained from the pigtail catheter placed above the native valve (see **Fig. 16**). THV delivery can then be performed after the steps described in the transfemoral approach section. After balloon deflation, the balloon delivery catheter is retrieved and the immediate results assessed by TEE before withdrawal of the guidewire. Repeat balloon

inflation is rarely needed. Post-THV aortography assesses the final result.

Final steps
The sheath is retrieved from the apex under manual compression, eventually during a brief episode of RVP to limit the risk of bleeding, and the puncture is closed using the purse-string

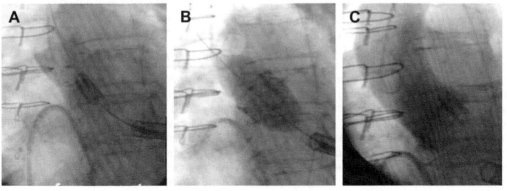

Fig. 16. Final phases of the transapical approach: (*A*) THV positioning across the native valve, (*B*) THV delivery under rapid pacing, (*C*) supra-aortic angiogram to assess the results post-THV delivery.

sutures. The chest wall is closed after insertion of a pleural chest drain and administration of protamine.

Postoperative care

Very early extubation is indicated in all possible cases, soon after transfer to the postoperative care unit. The same type of care as that after conventional cardiac surgery is required. In the absence of complication, patients are generally discharged after 6 to 8 days.

COMPLICATIONS

Complications of TAVI with the Edwards valve range from minor to potentially lethal adverse events. The learning curve plays an important role in the occurrence of complications, and their prevention, detection, and treatment do represent a crucial part of the Edwards training program. Even though vascular complications are more frequent with the transfemoral route, most other complications are common to the 2 approaches. Better understanding of these complications will continue to improve the clinical outcome.

Vascular Complications

Arterial injury does represent the more common complication associated with TAVI[20] and is mainly related to the large sheath size required for THV implantation. Careful patient screening with angiography and CT Scan imaging is the key to avoid these adverse events that can be directly or indirectly implicated to procedural mortality and impaired clinical outcome.[11]

The sheath must be removed as soon as the valve is deployed and its position corroborated. Sheath removal should be done after reinsertion of its dilator, while maintaining the stiff guidewire in place in the descending aorta, and with simultaneous contrast injection from the contralateral pigtail placed at the level of iliac bifurcation or an internal mammary catheter inserted into the iliac artery. If there is significant resistance, the sheath should not be pulled because the iliac or femoral artery may avulse completely. Covered stents and occlusion balloons should be available in the angiographic suite to treat arterial rupture. Arterial perforation can be life threatening and must be urgently treated by either covered stent or surgery, after transient balloon occlusion of the vessel proximal to the perforation. Flow-limiting dissections can be treated with noncovered stents, whereas complex arterial damage may require emergent arterial reconstruction. Angiography should always be performed after vessel repair to confirm vessel patency and runoff.

Traumatic aortic injury (aortic dissection, perforation, or rupture of the annulus) is rare and may require urgent management with balloon occlusion and conversion to thoracotomy for repair. However, in this population of very sick and elderly patients, severe aortic complications remain frequently fatal.

Stroke

Causes of stroke (0%–10%) are multiple,[8,10,20] potentially caused by plaque migration from the aortic arch or ascending aorta, migration of thrombus from the hardware, or mobilization of calcific material from the native valve during valve crossing, balloon inflation, or valve delivery or because of prolonged hypotension in patients with previous cerebrovascular disease. Lower stroke rates with the transapical approach have been reported. Management of hypotension and optimal anticoagulation are requested. Embolic protection devices may become soon available and could be useful in selected patients in the future.

THV Malpositioning and Embolization

Accurate positioning is the key to avoid coronary occlusion, mitral regurgitation, and permanent heart block. A too high or too low THV positioning may lead to paravalvular insufficiency due to a lack of apposition of the sealing cuff to the annulus. Placement of a second THV within the first one (valve in valve) may resolve the problem. Valve embolization can be the consequence of a malposition before delivery, suboptimal ventricular capture during RVP, or technical errors during THV deployment. THV embolization to the aorta can be easily managed by dragging the THV to the aortic arch or the descending aorta with a large-sized balloon inflated distally until an adequate landing zone is found. A second valve can then be placed in the native position. Embolization to the left ventricle is a much more serious event that requires conversion to thoracotomy for surgical ablation and subsequent AVR.

Perivalvular Regurgitation

Perivalvular AR may be caused by inappropriate valve position, valve underexpansion, or inappropriately sized valve. The vast majority of ARs are perivalvular, which can be confirmed by TTE or TEE. Postdilating the valve with a larger balloon is not often useful because the external cuff prevents overexpansion. Postdilating with the same volume can be done if the valve does not appear circular on fluoroscopy or TEE or if the full volume of contrast has not been administered during balloon inflation leading to suboptimal expansion. In very rare cases with severe AR related to THV valvular dysfunction, a second valve should be placed inside the new valve at the appropriate level. In general, perivalvular AR is well tolerated when mild to moderate,[8,11–15,20] and no hemolysis has been found at midterm follow-up.

Other Complications

Pericardial tamponade is a rare event and may be caused by heart perforation, most often of the right ventricle with the pacing lead that can often be managed by pericardiocentesis. Trauma of the left ventricle with the wires or delivery system is exceptional with the new-generation devices and may require surgical repair. Echocardiographic detection is mandatory in case of unexplained hypotension.

Coronary obstruction is exceptional. Coronary obstruction is exceptional and results, in most cases, in the displacement of a bulky calcific leaflet. This event can be predicted by detecting huge nodules on TTE, TEE, or CT Scan during the screening process and by supravalvular aortography in combination with balloon predilatation of the native valve. Successful management may require temporary cardiopulmonary support in association with percutaneous or surgical revascularization.[20,21]

Permanent pacemaker is required after TAVI in 3% to 12% of the cases[11–15] with the Edwards SAPIEN valve, a clearly lower rate than the 9% to 36% reported after CoreValve implantation.[22] It is related to injury of the atrioventricular conduction system by the THV, mainly in case of too low positioning within the outflow track. Transient (or permanent) heart block may also occur during balloon valvuloplasty or even valve crossing with the wire. Advanced age, massive subvalvular calcification, THV oversizing, or preexisting right bundle branch block are predisposing factors to complete heart block.[16]

Arrhythmias

Atrial fibrillation is more frequent with the transapical approach and may require cardioversion if the hemodynamics is compromised. Ventricular fibrillation may occur during intraventricular hardware manipulation or RVP and justifies the placement of defibrillator pads before the procedure.

Renal failure

In patients with renal failure, worsening of renal function may occur as the consequence of hypotension or contrast administration. Patient preparation and limitation of contrast volume are mandatory in these patients.

OVERVIEW OF RESULTS FROM THE LITERATURE

The procedural success, defined as a successful THV implantation without major complication, has consistently increased from 82% in the earliest transvenous experience[2,3] to 86% in the initial transarterial experience[5] and 93.8% in the recent Edwards SAPIEN Aortic Bioprosthesis European Outcome (SOURCE registry).[11] The success rate increases markedly with increasing experience.[8] Similarly, the complication rate and mortality at 30 days are steadily improving. In a review of 82 reports representing 2356 patients,[23] the 30-day survival was 89%, similar for both Edwards SAPIEN and CoreValve. In the most recent SOURCE registry,[11] 30-day survival was 91.2% and 81% at 1-year.

To put into perspective the state of the art with the Edwards SAPIEN valve, it is interesting to look at the recently reported results of the prospective pivotal PARTNER US randomized trial. In this trial, patients were randomly assigned to TAVI (transfemoral approach) versus medical treatment[14] in nonsurgical candidates (cohort B, 358 patients) or to TAVI versus AVR (cohort A, 699 patients) in high–surgical risk patients,[15] THV being implanted using either the transfemoral (244 patients) or the transapical route (104 patients) depending on the quality of the femoral access. The primary end point was the rate of death from any cause at 1 year. In cohort B, the superiority of TAVI over medical treatment was fully demonstrated. The death rate at 1 year was dramatically lower after TAVI than after medical treatment (30.7% vs 50.7%, P<.001), as well as the rate of cardiac symptoms (New York Heart Association class II or IV: 25.2% vs 58%, P<.001). In cohort A, the noninferiority of TAVI versus AVR was demonstrated. The death rate at 1 year was 24.2% versus 26.8%. Major vascular complications (11.0% vs 3.2% P<.001) and rate of major stroke at 1 year (5.1% vs 2.4%, P<.07) were more frequent after TAVI than after AVR, whereas major bleeding (9.3% vs 19.5%, P<.001) and new-onset atrial fibrillation (8.6% vs 16.0%, P<.001) were more frequent after AVR. Dramatic improvement of cardiac symptoms was similarly observed in the 2 groups at 1 year. This trial can definitely be considered a landmark for the future development of TAVI in nonsurgical and high–surgical risk patients with AS.

FUTURE DIRECTIONS

Even though TAVI was born 10 years ago, it remains a relatively new and rapidly evolving procedure for which its promising results explain its considerable acceptance and expansion world-wide. More than 300 centers are open in Europe to the Edwards' device, and the number of centers and investigators is steadily increasing. In the event of Food and Drug Administration approval, this technology might explode in the United States within a few months and might save the life of several nonsurgical patients there.

The Edwards SAPIEN valve has physical characteristics and hemodynamic performance similar to the latest generation of Edwards's surgical bioprosthesis. Even though little is known about the long-term results after Edwards SAPIEN TAVI, no evidence of structural valvular failure has been reported yet, and hemodynamics and favorable clinical outcome remain preserved at 3 years.[24] The selection of elderly and severely sick patients in all registries impairs the assessment of long-term results because longer outcome is determined primarily by comorbidities.[24] In the authors' experience, the longest follow-up has reached 6 years and a half, without any structural deterioration and with the persistence of excellent hemodynamics and clinical improvement. In the future, comprehensive registries and randomized trials would be necessary to better assess whether TAVI offers the same clinical benefit for the long term compared with surgical AVR in younger and less sick patients with AS.

The last generation of Edwards valve, the SAPIEN XT, available since 2010 in Europe, has dramatically improved and facilitated the technique of implantation. In comparison with the Edwards SAPIEN, this device presents with a cobalt chromium stent frame, an equal radial strength, and enhanced leaflets design. One of its main advantage is the reduced crimped profile compatible with 18F and 19F sheath sizes for the 23- and 26-mm valves, respectively. With this device, the transfemoral route can now be used in more than 70% of the cases, using a pure percutaneous approach with preclosing techniques. This new promising device is currently under investigation in the United States.

Other attractive investigational options are the use of the Edwards SAPIEN valve for the treatment of degenerated bioprosthesis (valve-in-valve) that has been shown safe and efficient for the treatment of aortic, pulmonary, mitral, and tricuspid prosthetic valve failures.[25]

SUMMARY

As expected from the early registries, TAVI with the Edwards SAPIEN valve has been shown to be highly beneficial to patients at high risk or with contraindications to surgical AVR. The availability of both transfemoral and transapical approaches allows the technique to be applied in the vast majority of patients. Optimal screening and technical proficiency are crucial for a successful and safe procedure. The technique poses many technical challenges in a cohort of very sick and fragile elderly patients that interventional cardiologists and surgeons are not used to treat. Thus, TAVI should remain confided to formally trained and proctored experienced physicians, in centers of expertise offering an optimal multidisciplinary collaboration.

At the price of an acceptable and decreasing rate of complications, the technique has been demonstrated to be lifesaving in patients who are not suitable candidates for surgery, whereas the mortality at 1 year and the improvement of symptoms are similar to AVR in high-risk patients. However, the long-term durability of the device remains to be determined before expanding the indications to younger and lower-risk patients with AS.

REFERENCES

1. Iung B, Baron G, Butchart EG, et al. A prospective survey of patients with valvular heart disease in Europe: the Euro Heart Survey on valvular heart disease. Eur Heart J 2003;24:1231–43.
2. Cribier A, Eltchaninoff H, Bash A, et al. Percutaneous transcatheter implantation of an aortic valve prosthesis for calcific aortic stenosis: first human case. Circulation 2002;106:3006–8.
3. Cribier A, Eltchaninoff H, Tron C, et al. Early experience with percutaneous transcatheter implantation of heart valve prosthesis for the treatment of end stage inoperable patients with calcific aortic stenosis. J Am Coll Cardiol 2004;43:698–703.
4. Cribier A, Eltchaninoff H, Tron C, et al. Treatment of calcific aortic stenosis with percutaneous heart valve. J Am Coll Cardiol 2006;47:1214–23.
5. Webb JG, Chandavimol M, Thompson CR, et al. Percutaneous aortic valve implantation retrograde from the femoral artery. Circulation 2006;113:842–50.
6. Webb JG, Pasupati S, Humphries K, et al. Percutaneous transarterial aortic valve replacement in selected high-risk patients with aortic stenosis. Circulation 2007;116:755–63.
7. Walther T, Falk V, Kempfert J, et al. Transapical minimally invasive aortic valve implantation: the initial 50 patients. Eur J Cardiothorac Surg 2008; 33:983–8.
8. Webb JG, Altwegg L, Boone RH, et al. Transcatheter aortic valve implantation: impact on clinical and valve-related outcomes. Circulation 2009;119:3009–16.
9. Rodes-Cabau J, Webb JG, Cheung A, et al. Transcatheter aortic valve implantation for the treatment

of severe symptomatic aortic stenosis in patients at very high or prohibitive risk; acute and late outcomes of the multicenter Canadian experience. J Am Coll Cardiol 2010;55:1080–90.

10. Walther T, Simon P, Dewey T, et al. Transapical minimally invasive aortic valve implantation: multicenter experience. Circulation 2007;116(Suppl 11):1240–5.

11. Thomas M, Schymik G, Walther T, et al. Thirty-day results of the SAPIEN Aortic Bioprosthesis European Outcome (SOURCE) registry of transcatheter aortic valve implantation using the Edwards SAPIEN valve. Circulation 2010;122:62–9.

12. Eltchaninoff H, Prat A, Gilard M, et al. Transcatheter aortic valve implantation: early results of the FRANCE (French Aortic National CoreValve and Edwards) registry. Eur Heart J 2011;32:191–7.

13. Lefevre T, Kappetein AP, Wolner E, et al. One year follow-up of the multi-centre European PARTNER transcatheter heart valve study. Eur Heart J 2011; 32:148–57.

14. Leon MB, Smith CR, Mack M, et al. Transcatheter aortic valve implantation in inoperable patients with severe aortic stenosis. N Engl J Med 2010;363:1587–607.

15. Smith CR, Leon MB, Mack MJ, et al. Transcatheter versus surgical aortic-valve replacement in high risk patients. N Engl J Med 2011;364:2187–607.

16. Godin M, Eltchaninoff H, Furuta A, et al. Frequency of conduction disturbances after transcatheter implantation of an Edwards Sapien aortic valve prosthesis. Am J Cardiol 2010;106:707–12.

17. Solomon LW, Fusman B, Jolly N, et al. Percutaneous suture closure for management of large French size arterial puncture in aortic valvuloplasty. J Invasive Cardiol 2001;13:592–6.

18. Agatiello C, Eltchaninoff H, Tron C, et al. Balloon aortic valvuloplasty in the adult. Immediate results and in-hospital complications in the latest series of 141 consecutive patients at the University Hospital of Rouen (2002-2005). Arch Mal Coeur Vaiss 2006; 99(3):195–200 [in French].

19. Webb JG, Pasupati S, Achtem L, et al. Rapid pacing to facilitate transcatheter prosthetic heart valve implantation. Catheter Cardiovasc Interv 2006;68: 199–204.

20. Masson LB, Kovak J, Schuler G, et al. Transcatheter aortic valve implantation: review of the nature, management and avoidance of procedural complications. JACC Cardiovasc Interv 2009;2:811–20.

21. Kapadia SR, Svensson L, Tuzcu EM. Successful percutaneous management of left main trunk occlusion during percutaneous aortic valve replacement. Catheter Cardiovasc Interv 2009;73:966–72.

22. Grube E, Buellesfeld L, Mueller R, et al. Progress and current status of percutaneous aortic valve replacement: results of three generations of the CoreValve Revalving System. Circ Cardiovasc Interv 2008;1:167–75.

23. Coeytaux RR, Williams JW, Gray RN, et al. Percutaneous heart valve replacement for aortic stenosis: state of the evidence. Ann Intern Med 2010;153: 314–24.

24. Gurvitch R, Wood DA, Tay EL, et al. Transcatheter aortic valve implantation. Durability of clinical and hemodynamic outcomes beyond 3 years in a large patient cohort. Circulation 2010;122:1319–27.

25. Webb JG, Wood DA, Gurvitch R, et al. Transcatheter valve-in-valve implantation for failed bioprosthetic heart valves. Circulation 2010;121:1848–57.

Transcatheter Aortic Valve Implantation: Experience with the CoreValve Device

Anita W. Asgar, MD, FRCPC, Raoul Bonan, MD*

KEYWORDS

- Transcatheter valve implantation • Medtronic CoreValve
- Self-expanding aortic valve

In the short time since the first implantation of a transcatheter aortic valve by Alain Cribier in 2002, the field of transcatheter aortic valve implantation has been rapidly evolving. The Medtronic CoreValve first emerged on the landscape in 2004 with initial first human studies, and it is currently being studied in the Pivotal US trial, which began enrolling in 2010. This article details the current experience with the self-expanding aortic valve with a focus on clinical results and ongoing challenges.

MEDTRONIC COREVALVE REVALVING SYSTEM

The Medtronic CoreValve Revalving system consists of the following 3 components: CoreValve bioprosthesis, the delivery catheter, and the disposable loading system.

The CoreValve bioprosthesis is a porcine pericardial valve sutured into a self-expandable nitinol frame. The nitinol frame is made of laser cut nitinol with diamond cells and a distinct funnel-like shape that measures between 5 and 355 mm in length. The frame has three distinct regions of radial force at the distal, middle and outflow portion of the device. The distal portion of the device has high radial force to maintain intra-annular anchoring, and it is covered with a pericardial skirt to minimize paravalvular aortic regurgitation. The middle portion is constrained at the level of the porcine pericardial leaflets, and

it is designed to avoid impingement of the coronary arteries while providing supra-annular leaflet function. The outflow portion of the prosthesis has low radial force and provides a means of orienting the device in the ascending aorta (**Fig. 1**). The valve leaflets are composed of six separate segments of porcine pericardium that are sutured to the frame in a supra-annular position. The supra-annular position reduces leaflet stress and optimizes leaflet motion.[1] In addition, it ensures optimal valve function despite inadequate frame expansion as described by Jilaihawi and colleagues.[2]

The delivery catheter has undergone numerous iterations since its inception. The first-generation device was a 25 French (Fr) catheter. The second-generation device studied in the safety and efficacy trial was 21Fr followed by the third-generation 18Fr device, which consists of the 18 Fr capsule, which houses the valve and a 12Fr shaft. The current delivery system being used in the US randomized trial has also incorporated a 15Fr stability layer on the delivery system, called Accutrak (Medtronic, Minneapolis, MN, USA), which isolates the retractable delivery sheath from the introducer to provide a stable platform for valve delivery.

The valve is loaded onto the delivery catheter and then deployed by removing the capsule; once in position in the left ventricular outflow tract, the delivery catheter is withdrawn, and the valve self-expands into place. The valve deployment is

Montreal Heart Institute, 5000 Belanger, Montreal H1T1C8, Quebec, Canada
* Corresponding author.
E-mail address: raoul.bonan@mmic.net

Intervent Cardiol Clin 1 (2012) 27–36
doi:10.1016/j.iccl.2011.09.005
2211-7458/12/$ – see front matter © 2012 Elsevier Inc. All rights reserved.

interventional.theclinics.com

A

Outflow Portion

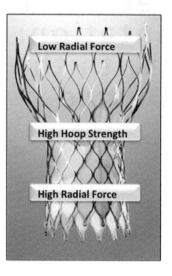

1. Sits in ascending aorta
2. Provides PAV alignment

Constrained Portion
(with valve leaflets)

1. Supra-annular leaflet function
2. Designed to avoid coronaries

Inflow Portion
(with skirt)

1. Intra-annular anchoring
2. Conforms to native annulus
3. Minimizes paravalvular aortic regurgitation

Low Radial Force

High Hoop Strength

High Radial Force

B

- No rapid pacing required
- Physician can take time to deploy properly
- Can adjust valve position through the procedure
- Can witness valve function before releasing

- No trauma to the valve leaflet from a balloon

Ease of use is critical to procedural success

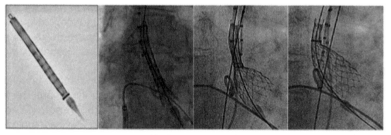

Fig. 1. (A) Percutaneous aortic valve design, 3 levels. (B) Self-expanding frame leads to superior ease of use and potentially better outcomes.

slow and controlled, and device position can be adjusted during deployment. The device is currently available in 22 sizes, 26 mm and 29 mm to treat an annulus of 20 to 23 mm and 24 to 27 mm respectively, with a 31 mm device currently in development.

EARLY CLINICAL EXPERIENCE

The first-in-man series of patients treated with the CoreValve revalving system was performed in Sieburg, Germany. Twenty-five high-risk patients with symptomatic severe aortic patients and contraindications for surgery were enrolled in the single-center registry. Patients were treated with the first- (24Fr) and second- (21Fr) generation Core-Valve devices. Device and procedural success were achieved in 88% and 84% of patients, and

18 patients survived to hospital discharge. Mean aortic valve gradient improved from 44 to 12 mm Hg with a corresponding improvement in functional class. This study demonstrated the feasibility of aortic valve replacement with a self-expanding device and also highlighted some of the procedural challenges including thrombocytopenia requiring pretreatment with clopidogrel and device positioning.[3]

Thirty-day clinical outcomes with the second- and third-generation CoreValve prosthesis in 86 patients confirmed feasibility in high-risk patients and demonstrated a lower than predicted procedural mortality in these high-risk patients of 6%. Overall 30-day mortality was 12%, with a combined rate of death, stroke, and myocardial infarction of 22%. The use of the 18Fr device mitigated the requirement for surgical cutdown in almost half of patients. In addition, fewer patients with the 18Fr system underwent the procedure with hemodynamic support. Hemodynamic results were good, with a decrease in aortic valve gradient and an increase in valve area that were sustained at 30 days. Functional class was also improved, with a decline in New York Heart Association Class of 2.85 before to 1.85 after valve implantation.[4]

CURRENT CLINICAL EXPERIENCE

In May 2007, the CoreValve revaling system received CE Mark approval, and the technology became available for the treatment of high-risk aortic stenosis patients in Europe. Since that time, over 12,000 implants have been performed worldwide. Such widespread adoption of the technology has resulted in increased operator experience, higher procedural success, and the recognition of new challenges. A summary of published data is presented in **Table 1** and **Fig. 2**.

Cardiac conduction system abnormalities are not uncommon in patients with aortic valvestenosis, and surgical aortic valve replacement has been associated with the requirement of a permanent pacemaker in 3% to 8% of patients, in part due to the proximity of the conduction system to the aortic valve. Initial case reports had highlighted an increased incidence of conduction anomalies after transcatheter aortic valve implantation (TAVI), and this was further described by a retrospective study that demonstrated apossible link between positioning of the Medtronic CoreValve and the incidence of left bundle branch block (LBBB) and subsequent pacemakers.[5] The exact mechanism of conduction system anomalies is unclear, but there are numerous theories. Given the proximity of the atrioventricular node and left bundle to the aortic valve and left ventricular outflow tract, the depth of prosthesis implant may have an effect. A retrospective study of 70 patients undergoing TAVI identified depth of implant and pre-existing right bundle branch block as potential risk factors for permanent pacemaker implantation.[6] Other theories include the volume of calcification of the device landing zone, which may create a mass effect or pressure on the conduction system in that region after device-deployment.[7] Interestingly, other work has demonstrated that LBBB often develops after balloon valvuloplasty, suggesting perhaps a traumatic etiology that occurs before valve implantation that may be related to oversizing of the balloon with respect to the aortic annulus.[8] Although plausible, this does not explain the relatively lower incidence of permanent pacemakers required in those patients receiving the Edwards device (Edwards LifeScience, Irvine, CA,

USA), which is balloon-expandable and requires a minimum of 2 balloon dilatations rather than one.

Two-year follow-up data from the third-generation safety and efficacy trial were published in 2011. These data included 126 patients treated with the 18Fr CoreValve revaling system from 2006 to 2008 in Europe and Canada. Procedural success was modest, 83%; however, this was relatively early in the overall experience with the technology, and 30-day mortality was 15.2%. At 2-year follow up, all-cause mortality was 38.1%, and permanent pacemakers were required in 26.2% of patients for atrioventricular conduction abnormalities. There was no evidence of deterioration in the hemodynamic result during the 2-year follow up, and improvements in functional class were also maintained. Importantly, this study illustrated the durability of the transcatheter Medtronic CoreValve at a minimum of 2 years.[9]

The largest published series of patients treated with the third-generation CoreValve revaling system, an Italian multicenter study, had high rates of procedural success with low procedural mortality, 98% and 0.9%, respectively in this high-risk elderly population. This series identified factors predictive of mortality including conversion to open heart surgery, cardiac tamponade, major access complications, and low ejection fraction. Of note, the highest mortality was observed within the first 2 weeks following the procedure, often related to procedural complications. Mortality continued at a steady rate in this population of 0.9% per month during the first year as result of patient comorbidities, for a 1-year mortality rate of 15%. The rate of vascular access complications was low, 2%, and the need for a permanent pacemaker was 17.4% at 30 days.[10]

ALTERNATIVE ACCESS SITES

Transfemoral access for retrograde transcatheter aortic valve implantation has been the access route of choice for the majority of high-risk patients with severe aortic stenosis. This elderly group of patients is often plagued with peripheral vascular disease that makes the transfemoral procedure difficult. Transapical valve implantation using the Edwards device has been performed successfully; however, this route requires a thoracotomy, which can be associated with significant morbidity. Subclavian or transaxillary access using the Medtronic CoreValve as well as direct aortic access has become alternatives to femoral access in this particular patient group (**Fig. 3**A, B).

Early reports with the transaxillary approach demonstrated its feasibility as a route for transcatheter aortic valve implantation.[11,12] The

Table 1
Summary of published results of the Medtronic CoreValve

Reference	Study	Year of Publication	Number of Patients	Mean Age	Mean EuroScore	Procedural Success	30-day Mortality	Stroke	Vascular Complications	Permanent Pacemaker	Follow-up	Mortality at Follow-up	Mean Aortic Gradient at Follow-up
20	Belgian registry	2011	141	82 ± 6	25 ± 15	98%	11%	4%	NA	22%	1 year	21.00%	—
9	18Fr SE trial	2011	126	82	23.40	83.10%	15.20%	9.60%	NA	26.20%	2 years	38.10%	9.0 ± 3.4 mm Hg
21	Germany	2011	51	78 ± 6	19.6 ± 11.3	98%	10%	NA	11.40%	40%	1 year	16%	NA
10	Italian registry	2011	663	81 ± 7	23 ± 13.7	98%	5.40%	1.20%	2.00%	16.60%	1 year	15%	10 ± 4.9 mm Hg
22	Switzerland	2011	140	83 ± 5	24.5 ± 16	95.40%	6.20%	4.60%	11.50%	26.90%	30 days	6.20%	8.4 ± 4.2 mm Hg
23	Netherlands	2011	165	81 ± 8	13.1		9.70%	6.70%	15%	17.50%	30 days	9.70%	NA
24	France	2011	78	82.3 ± 7	24.7 ± 11.2	92.60%	14.10%	4.50%	7.50%	25.70%	30 days	14.10%	NA

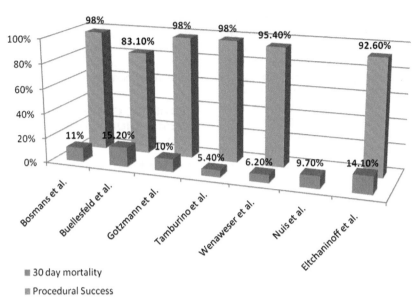

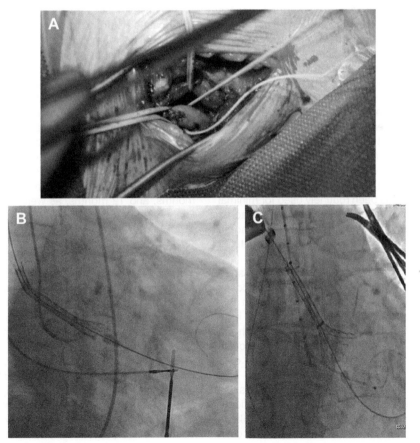

Fig. 2. Procedural success and 30-day mortality in published clinical experience of the Medtronic CoreValve. (*Data from* Refs.[9,10,20–24])

Fig. 3. (*A*) Surgical approach of the sub-clavian artery. (*B*) Xray imaging of a sub-clavian implantation. (*C*) Xray imaging of a direct aortic implantation.

approach has advantages over the traditional femoral approach; the shorter distance between the annulus and the catheter provides greater control during valve positioning and delivery. From a surgical perspective, the access is straight-forward, and the artery is rarely severely diseased even in the elderly population (see **Fig. 3**A, B). A case series of 17 patients undergoing TAVI via the subclavian artery illustrated that the procedure could be performed safely with no subclavian artery injury. Most cases were performed from the left subclavian artery, including 2 patients with previous left internal mammary artery (LIMA) grafts. Although there were no complications in these cases, caution should likely be exercised, as dissection of the subclavian may have dire consequences for those patients dependant on LIMA graft flow.[13]

A direct comparison of transfemoral and subclavian TAVI performed in the United Kingdom in 288 consecutive patients revealed that subclavian patients were higher risk according to Logistic Euroscore estimates, and were more likely to have carotid disease in addition to peripheral vascular disease. In this cohort of 35 patients treated by subclavian access, procedural success was obtained in 100% of cases, with higher rates of optimal positioning and lower rates of major vascular complications. Interestingly, despite having higher rates of cerebrovascular disease, the subclavian group did not have a higher incidence of stroke.[14] These results were consistent with those seen in 54 TAVI patients treated via the subclavian artery in Italy.[15]

In addition to the subclavian approach for TAVI, direct aortic access is emerging as another option for patients with severe peripheral vascular disease. This technique uses a right anterior thoracotomy, which has been routinely used for minimal invasive aortic valve replacement. The direct aortic approach provides direct access to the aortic annulus, and the proximity to the valve facilitates manipulation and delivery of the device (see **Fig. 3**C). Bruschi and colleagues[16] have published a series of 6 patients with the direct aortic access for TAVI using the Medtronic CoreValve. In this series, procedural access was achieved in 5 cases, all of whom were discharged with an improvement in functional class and evidence of hemodynamic improvement at a follow-up of 6 months.

The quest for alternate access sites is an important one, as many patients have significant peripheral vascular disease. Currently available technology for TAVI includes transapical access for patients with ileofemoral disease; however, this technique is not without its challenges, and

recent data suggest that the trend is toward less favorable outcomes than with conventional surgery.[17] The availability of a subclavian and direct aortic access provides another option in the management of such patients.

MEDTRONIC COREVALVE US INVESTIGATIONAL DEVICE EXEMPTION TRIAL DESIGN

The Medtronic CoreValve US investigational device exemption (IDE) trial started at the end of 2010 with the purpose of evaluating the safety and efficacy of the Medtronic CoreValve system in the treatment of symptomatic severe aortic stenosis in subjects needing aortic valve replacement (**Fig. 4**). Two cohorts of patients will be studied; an extreme-risk cohort with a predicted operative mortality or serious, irreversible morbidity risk estimated at greater than or equal to 50% at 30 days, and a high-risk cohort with an expected perioperative mortality estimated at 15% (based on investigator estimated mortality or Society of Thoracic Surgery (STS) score >10). The extreme-risk cohort will be followed in a prospective registry for the composite endpoint of all-cause death or major stroke, with a sample size of 487 iliofemoral subjects and up to 100 non-iliofemoral subjects in the United States. The High-risk cohort will be randomized in a one-to-one fashion against conventional surgery surgical aortic valve replacement (SAVR) with a primary endpoint of all-cause death or major stroke at 12 months. The randomized trial will be conducted at up to 45 sites in the United States, with a sample size of 790 subjects (395 Medtronic CoreValve System TAVI and 395 SAVR) with a follow-up through 5 years with assessments at 30 days, 6 months, and 12 months, as well as 2, 3, 4 and 5 years.

ONGOING CHALLENGES

Now that the feasibility and effectiveness of transcatheter valve implantation has been established, the focus has begun to shift to the ongoing challenges with this technology, namely reducing complications. Data from the completed Placement of AoRTic TraNscathetER Valve Trial (PARTNER) have highlighted important issues with regards to stroke in the patient population undergoing TAVI, with rates of major stroke as high as 5% to 8%.[17] Studies of patients undergoing TAVI with the Edwards device have also confirmed the presence of new cerebral lesions on magnetic resonance imaging (MRI) after procedure even in asymptomatic patients.[18] Published

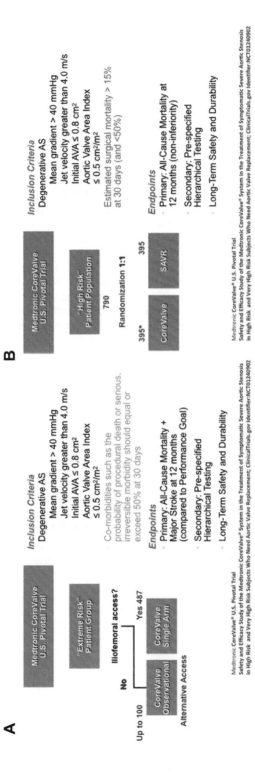

Fig. 4. (A) CoreValve US Pivotal Trial, extreme-risk study. (B) CoreValve US Pivotal Trial, high-risk study.

A

Medtronic CoreValve
U.S. Pivotal Trial

"Extreme Risk"
Patient Group

Iliofemoral access?

No   Yes 487

Up to 100

CoreValve
Observational   CoreValve
Single Arm

Alternative Access

Inclusion Criteria
- Degenerative AS
  - Mean gradient > 40 mmHg
  - Jet velocity greater than 4.0 m/s
  - Initial AVA ≤ 0.8 cm²
  - Aortic Valve Area Index
    ≤ 0.5 cm²/m²
- Co-morbidities such as the probability of procedural death or serious, irreversible morbidity should equal or exceed 50% at 30 days

Endpoints
- Primary: All-Cause Mortality + Major Stroke at 12 months (compared to Performance Goal)
- Secondary: Pre-specified Hierarchical Testing
- Long-Term Safety and Durability

Medtronic CoreValve® U.S. Pivotal Trial
Safety and Efficacy Study of the Medtronic CoreValve® System in the Treatment of Symptomatic Severe Aortic Stenosis
in High Risk and Very High Risk Subjects Who Need Aortic Valve Replacement; ClinicalTrials.gov Identifier:NCT01240902

B

Medtronic CoreValve
U.S. Pivotal Trial

"High Risk"
Patient Population

790

Randomization 1:1

395*   395

CoreValve   SAVR

Inclusion Criteria
- Degenerative AS
  - Mean gradient > 40 mmHg
  - Jet velocity greater than 4.0 m/s
  - Initial AVA ≤ 0.8 cm²
  - Aortic Valve Area Index
    ≤ 0.5 cm²/m²
- Estimated surgical mortality > 15% at 30 days (and <50%)

Endpoints
- Primary: All-Cause Mortality at 12 months (non-inferiority)
- Secondary: Pre-specified Hierarchical Testing
- Long-Term Safety and Durability

Medtronic CoreValve® U.S. Pivotal Trial
Safety and Efficacy Study of the Medtronic CoreValve® System in the Treatment of Symptomatic Severe Aortic Stenosis
in High Risk and Very High Risk Subjects Who Need Aortic Valve Replacement; ClinicalTrials.gov Identifier:NCT01240902

data from various centers using the Medtronic-CoreValve have published stroke rates from 2% to 8%; however, definitions are variable, and most did not include MRI in all patients (see **Table 1**). The exact mechanism of stroke has yet to be defined; however, embolic phenomenon is most likely. Various embolic protection devices are currently under investigation and may eventually play a permanent role in these procedures if they can demonstrate a reduction in events (**Fig. 5**). The late neurologic events are less well understood; could the etiology be related to platelet activation as a result of the stent or micro emboli? Further work is required, and much will rest on the current ongoing randomized controlled trial of the Medtronic CoreValve.

Vascular access complications also remain an area of consideration for TAVI. The PARTNER trial and registry data have illustrated that vascular access complications are associated with higher mortality and worse prognosis.[17] Currently available devices are 18Fr; however, in the elderly population, transfemoral vascular access remains challenging as a result of comorbidities and in the absence of reliable closure devices. The development of large bore closure devices is

fervently underway, and alternative access sites have also gained popularity. However, this issue remains and will need to be addressed as the technology matures.

The need for permanent pacemakers in patients after CoreValve was an unexpected finding, as previously discussed, and will need to be better understood as the technology permeates to the younger age groups. Current pacemaker rates after procedure range form 10% to 25%; however, the indications have been nebulous in many studies. Data from the US Pivotal trial will undoubtedly shed more light on this subject.

As speculation begins on the expansion of this technology to a younger patient population at lower surgical risk, the issue of paravalvular regurgitation will need to be addressed. Data from the United Kingdom from 2007 to 2009, documented the prevalence of paravalvular regurgitation at 1 year to be 77%; 54% had less than mild regurgitation and 34% greater than mild regurgitation (**Fig. 6**).[19] No patient had severe paravalvular aortic regurgitation (AR). The regurgitation is predominantly seen in the area of the fibrous trigone of the heart as a result of a nonconformity between the base of the device and the aortic

A

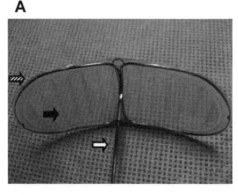

B

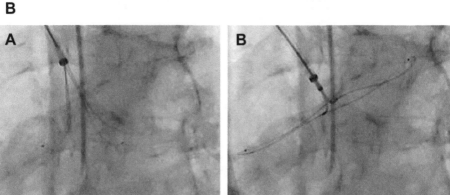

Fig. 5. (*A*) Picture of the Embolic Protection Device; (*B*) (*A*) Xray imaging of the device during deployment (*B*) Device fully deployed in position.

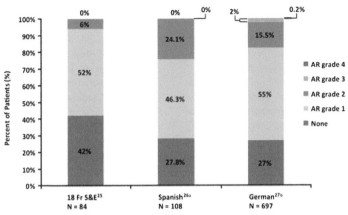

Fig. 6. Postprocedure aortic regurgitation. [a]Measured with angiography. [b]German registry data include both patients treated with CoreValve, 84.5% and EDW Sapien, 15.5%. (*Data from* Refs.[25–27])

annulus. In addition, the magnitude and localization of aortic leaflet and annular calcification may also play a role in paravalvular AR. In the future, an adequate match between the aortic annulus and the device may be part of the solution. Despite a worldwide experience that spans several years, the anatomic effects of implantation of the Medtronic CoreValve are not entirely understood, in particular the interaction of the device with the aortic root, annulus, and left ventricle outflow tract (LVOT). Transforming the 3 axes; aortic root, aortic annulus, and LVOT, into one with the CoreValve may create tension in the adjacent tissues and ventricular septum that may result in conduction system abnormalities and malapposition with the aortic annulus resulting in paravalvular leaks.

The field of transcatheter valve implantation is still in its infancy; however, with one randomized trial already completed, the Medtronic CoreValve trial already underway, and over 12,000 patients treated worldwide, it is evolving rapidly. There are many unanswered questions; however, with science as the guide and thoughtful clinicians to light the way, the road ahead looks very promising.

REFERENCES

1. Grube E, Laborde JC, Zickmann B, et al. First report on a human percutaneous transluminal implantation of a self-expanding valve prosthesis for interventional treatment of aortic valve stenosis. Catheter Cardiovasc Interv 2005;66(4):465–9.

2. Jilaihawi H, Asgar A, Bonan R. Good outcome and valve function despite Medtronic CoreValve underexpansion. Catheter Cardiovasc Interv 2010;76(7): 1022–5.

3. Grube E, Laborde JC, Gerckens U, et al. Percutaneous implantation of the CoreValve self-expanding valve prosthesis in high-risk patients with aortic valve

disease: the Siegburg first-in-man study. Circulation 2006;114(15):1616–24.

4. Grube E, Schuler G, Buellesfeld L, et al. Percutaneous aortic valve replacement for severe aortic stenosis in high-risk patients using the second- and current third-generation self-expanding CoreValve prosthesis. J Am Coll Cardiol 2007;50(1): 69–76.

5. Piazza N, Onuma Y, Jesserun E, et al. Early and persistent intraventricular conduction abnormalities and requirements for pacemaking after percutaneous replacement of the aortic valve. JACC Cardiovasc Interv 2008;1(3):310–6.

6. Fraccaro C, Buja G, Tarantini G, et al. Incidence, predictors, and outcome of conduction disorders after transcatheter self-expandable aortic valve implantation. Am J Cardiol 2011;107(5):747–54.

7. Latsios G, Gerckens U, Buellesfeld L, et al. Device landing zone calcification, assessed by MSCT, as a predictive factor for pacemaker implantation after TAVI. Catheter Cardiovasc Interv 2010;76(3):431–9.

8. Nuis RJ, Van Mieghem NM, Schultz CJ, et al. Timing and potential mechanisms of new conduction abnormalities during the implantation of the Medtronic CoreValve System in patients with aortic stenosis. Eur Heart J 2011;32(16):2067–74.

9. Buellesfeld L, Gerckens U, Schuler G, et al. 2-year follow-up of patients undergoing transcatheter aortic valve implantation using a self-expanding valve prosthesis. J Am Coll Cardiol 2011;57(16):1650–7.

10. Tamburino C, Capodanno D, Ramondo A, et al. Incidence and predictors of early and late mortality after transcatheter aortic valve implantation in 663 patients with severe aortic stenosis. Circulation 2011;123(3):299–308.

11. Asgar A, Mullen MJ, Delahunty N, et al. Transcatheter aortic valve intervention through the axillary artery for the treatment of severe aortic stenosis. J Thorac Cardiovasc Surg 2009;137(3):773–5.

12. Fraccaro C, Napodano M, Tarantini G, et al. Expanding the eligibility for transcatheter aortic valve implantationthe trans-subclavian retrograde approach using the III generation CoreValve revalving system. JACC Cardiovasc Interv 2009;2(9):828–33.

13. Modine T, Obadia JF, Choukroun E, et al. Transcutaneous aortic valve implantation using the axillary/subclavian access: feasibility and early clinical outcomes. J Thorac Cardiovasc Surg 2011;141(2). 487–91.e1.

14. Moynagh AM, Scott DJ, Baumbach A, et al. CoreValve transcatheter aortic valve implantation via the subclavian arterycomparison with the transfemoral approach. J Am Coll Cardiol 2011;57(5):634–5.

15. Petronio AS, De Carlo M, Bedogni F, et al. Safety and efficacy of the subclavian approach for transcatheter aortic valve implantation with the CoreValve revalving system. Circ Cardiovasc Interv 2010;4:359–66.

16. Bruschi G, De Marco F, Fratto P, et al. Alternative approaches for transcatheter self-expanding aortic bioprosthetic valves implantation: single-center experience. Eur J Cardiothorac Surg 2011;39(6): e151–8.

17. Smith C, Leon MB, Mack MJ, et al. Transcatheter versus surgical aortic valve replacement in high-risk patients. N Engl J Med 2011;364(23):2187–98.

18. Rodés-Cabau J, Dumont E, Boone RH, et al. Cerebral embolism following transcatheter aortic valve implantation: comparison of transfemoral and transapical approaches. J Am Coll Cardiol 2011;57(1): 18–28.

19. Rajani R, Kakad M, Khawaja MZ, et al. Paravalvular regurgitation one year after transcatheter aortic valve implantation. Catheter Cardiovasc Interv 2010;75(6):868–72.

20. Bosmans JM, Kefer J, De Bruyne B, et al. Procedural, 30-day and one year outcome following CoreValve or Edwards transcatheter aortic valve implantation: results of the Belgian national registry. Interact Cardiovasc Thorac Surg 2011;12(5):762–7.

21. Gotzmann M, Bojara W, Lindstaedt M, et al. One-year results of transcatheter aortic valve implantation in severe symptomatic aortic valve stenosis. Am J Cardiol 2011;107(11):1687–92.

22. Wenaweser P, Pilgrim T, Roth N, et al. Clinical outcome and predictors for adverse events after transcatheter aortic valve implantation with the use of different devices and access routes. Am Heart J 2011;161(6):1114–24.

23. Nuis RJ, van Mieghem NM, van der Boon RM, et al. Effect of experience on results of transcatheter aortic valve implantation using a Medtronic CoreValve system. Am J Cardiol 2011;107(12):1824–9.

24. Eltchaninoff H, Prat A, Gilard M, et al. Transcatheter aortic valve implantation: early results of the FRANCE (FRench Aortic National CoreValve and Edwards) registry. Eur Heart J 2011;32:191–7.

25. Gerckens U. Safety, durability, and effectiveness at two years with the 18 Fr CoreValve transcatheter aortic valve. Paris: EuroPCR; 2010.

26. Avanzas P, Munoz-Garcia AJ, Segura J, et al. Percutaneous implantation of the CoreValve self-expanding aortic valve prosthesis in patients with severe aortic stenosis: early experience in Spain. Rev Esp Cardiol 2010;63:141–8.

27. Zahn R. German Registry, TAVI Facts, figures and national registries. Paris: EuroPCR; 2010.

Transcatheter Aortic Valve Implantation: Upcoming New Devices

Jan-Malte Sinning, MD, Nikos Werner, MD,
Georg Nickenig, MD, Eberhard Grube, MD*

KEYWORDS

- Aortic stenosis • CoreValve • Edwards-SAPIEN
- Embolic protection • Periprosthetic regurgitation • TAVI

Inspired by the first percutaneous transcatheter pulmonary valve replacement,[1] the first transcatheter heart valve implantation in the aortic position via trans-septal access with a balloon-expandable prosthesis was performed in 2002.[2] In 2005, the first self-expandable transcatheter aortic valve was implanted via retrograde passage of the aortic valve.[3]

Since then, more than 40,000 transcatheter aortic valve prostheses have been implanted worldwide. Transcatheter aortic valve implantation (TAVI) has been established as an alternative to surgical aortic valve replacement (SAVR) for patients with symptomatic severe aortic stenosis and high or prohibitive operative risk.[4,5] The PARTNER (Placement of Aortic Transcatheter Valve) trial was the first randomized controlled trial to show that TAVI is not only superior to conservative management in inoperable patients but also is equivalent to SAVR in high-risk patients, with similar rates of survival at 1 year.

According to the German TAVI registry, approximately one-third of all aortic valve prostheses in 2011 will be transcatheter heart valves.[6] Among cardiac surgeons, a trend toward the use of bioprosthetic heart valves has been noted: younger patients are more frequently treated with a surgical

bioprosthetic heart valve, because these valves might be treated by valve-in-valve implantation with transcatheter heart valves in case of degeneration and patients do not necessarily have to undergo repeat surgery. Thus, patients are able to do without life-long, oral anticoagulation.

Although the PARTNER trial recently underscored the value of TAVI for high-risk patients, with similar outcomes compared with SAVR, important differences in periprocedural risks and several TAVI-associated drawbacks have been identified, which should be addressed before the use of TAVI can be extended to younger and healthier patients. These drawbacks include, for example, the occurrence of periprocedural and postprocedural stroke but also the higher incidence of vascular complications, conduction disturbances, and periprosthetic aortic regurgitation after TAVI compared with SAVR. Upcoming devices will focus on these issues to optimize the outcome after TAVI.

PERIPROSTHETIC AORTIC REGURGITATION

Up to 40% of all patients after SAVR have trace or mild periprosthetic aortic regurgitation; approximately 5% suffer from moderate or severe

Disclosure: Dr Eberhard Grube is a proctor for CoreValve/Medtronic. The other authors report no conflicts of interest.
Medizinische Klinik und Poliklinik II, Universitätsklinikum Bonn, Rheinische Friedrich-Wilhelms-Universität, Sigmund-Freud-Street 25, Bonn 53105, Germany
* Corresponding author.
E-mail address: GrubeE@aol.com

Intervent Cardiol Clin 1 (2012) 37–43
doi:10.1016/j.iccl.2011.09.002

periprosthetic aortic regurgitation.[7] In TAVI, para-valvular leaks occur in 50% to 70% of all patients.[8] 15% to 20% of all TAVI patients suffer from moderate or severe periprosthetic aortic regurgitation after the procedure, independent of valve type and access route.[5,8–11]

The self-expanding Medtronic CoreValve Re-Valving System (Medtronic, Minneapolis, MN, USA) will soon be available in 4 sizes (23, 26, 29, and 31 mm) for annulus diameters from 18 to 29 mm (**Fig. 1**A). The balloon-expandable Edwards-SAPIEN XT valve prosthesis (Edwards Lifesciences, Irvine, CA, USA) is now available in 3 different sizes for the treatment of annulus diameters from 18 to 27 mm (see **Fig. 1**B). Because oversizing plays a pivotal role for the fixation of transcatheter

heart valves in the annulus of the native valve, implantation depth and prosthesis size are essential to reduce the rate and the severity of periprosthetic aortic regurgitation. Thus, larger prosthesis sizes improve postprocedural results in patients with a borderline annulus. If the stent frame of the valve is not fully expanded because of heavily calcified cusps of the native aortic valve, a postdilation with balloon valvuloplasty helps to reduce periprosthetic aortic regurgitation in most cases.

Next-generation Transcatheter Heart Valves

Repositionable and recapturable transcatheter heart valves will provide another step toward optimal positioning of the prosthesis and prevention

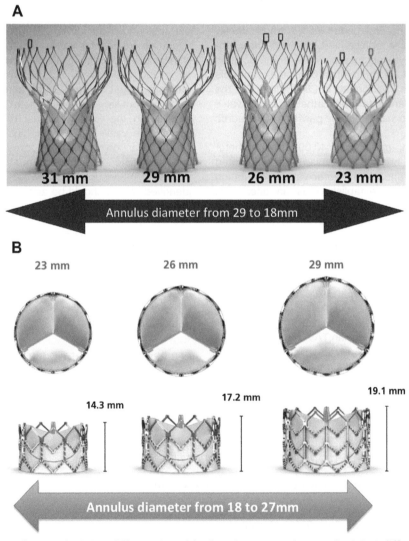

Fig. 1. (*A*) CoreValve prosthesis in 4 different sizes. (*B*) Edwards-SAPIEN valve prosthesis in 3 different sizes. ([*A*] *Courtesy of* Medtronic, Minneapolis, MN; with permission. [*B*] *Courtesy of* Edwards Lifesciences, Irvine, CA; with permission.)

of paravalvular leaks with consecutive periprosthetic aortic regurgitation.

The Sadra Medical Lotus valve (Boston Scientific, Natick, MA, USA) is one of these next-generation transcatheter heart valves. The Sadra Aortic Valve prosthesis consists of a trileaflet bovine pericardial tissue valve mounted on a self-expanding nitinol stent frame. The prosthesis is positioned over a three-armed system that allows a controlled deployment with the possibility of repositioning the valve in case of clinically significant periprosthetic aortic regurgitation (**Fig. 2**). An additional so-called adaptive seal at the lower part of the prosthesis skirt helps to further reduce periprosthetic aortic regurgitation by filling the gap between prosthesis and the annulus of the native valve.

The Direct Flow Medical aortic valve is a repositionable and recapturable prosthesis (Direct Flow Medical, Santa Rosa, CA, USA). The prosthesis consists of a bovine pericardial tissue valve that is mounted between 2 inflatable polyester rings. These 2 rings are able to adapt to the native aortic annulus and the left ventricular outflow tract to prevent periprosthetic aortic regurgitation. The device is deployed over an 18-French catheter-based, four-armed system into the annulus of the native aortic valve (**Fig. 3**A and B). To better visualize the prosthesis under fluoroscopy for an optimal positioning, the polyester rings of the prosthesis are filled with a mix of saline and contrast dye. Before final deployment of the valve, this fluid is exchanged against a hardening medium to firmly anchor the prosthesis in the native annulus (see **Fig. 3**C). If necessary, the rings can be fully deflated and the valve prosthesis can be retrieved with a net basket (see **Fig. 3**D).

VASCULAR COMPLICATIONS

To reduce the rate of major vascular complications, which were observed significantly more often in TAVI patients than in SAVR patients despite surgical closure of the access site (11.3% vs 3.5%)[5] in the PARTNER trial cohort A, diameters of the current devices have been reduced and new access routes have been established.

Transfemoral Approach

An inflatable sheath (Onset Medical Corp, Irvine, CA, USA) is available for the transfemoral approach with both commercially available TAVI devices and a shorter device for access via the subclavian artery. The uninflated sheath has a diameter of 13 French and is dilated to an external diameter of 19 to 21 French (depending on the prosthesis used) after introduction into the access vessel. In the near future, a recollapsible/deflatable sheath will be available that might be even more atraumatic.

In addition, the expandable eSheath from Edwards has been launched this year. The eSheath has an external diameter of 16 French for the 23-mm prosthesis and of 18 French for the 26-mm prosthesis. This flexible sheath only expands during introduction and advancement of the valve prosthesis through the sheath and, thus, might also be more atraumatic than a standard sheath. In addition, together with the new Nova-Flex Plus catheter system from Edwards Lifesciences, the eSheath makes it possible to retrieve the unexpanded valve prosthesis.

Alternative Access Routes

For transapical use, the Medtronic Engager aortic valve prosthesis is an alternative to the existing Edwards-SAPIEN system.[12] This valve has been used in a registered trial and will be launched soon. The valve has a trileaflet bovine pericardial tissue design mounted on a self-expanding nitinol stent frame that is covered with a polyester skirt to prevent periprosthetic aortic regurgitation (**Fig. 4**). In addition, this prosthesis for transapical use has a low device implant height to ensure clearance from coronary ostia and positioning arms that are anchored over the native leaflets to make an optimal alignment of the valve in the native annulus

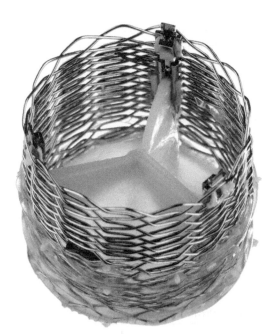

Fig. 2. Next-generation transcatheter heart valve I: Sadra Medical Lotus valve. (*Courtesy of* Sadra Medical/Boston Scientific, Natick, MA; with permission.)

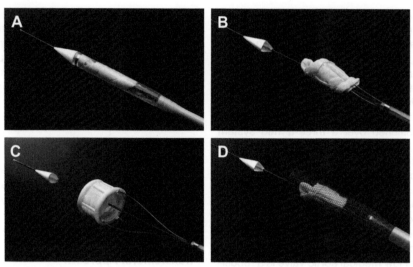

Fig. 3. Next-generation transcatheter heart valve II: Direct Flow Medical aortic valve. Valve loaded in deployment catheter (*A*). Deflated valve (*B*). Inflated valve with 4-armed steering device for an optimal positioning of the valve prosthesis during the TAVI procedure (*C*). Deflated valve prosthesis in retrieval basket (*D*). (*Courtesy of* Direct Flow Medical, Santa Rosa, CA; with permission.)

possible and, thus, to prevent periprosthetic aortic regurgitation.

The mortality risk associated with the transapical access route seems to be slightly higher compared with transfemoral access, as recently observed in the PARTNER EU trial.[13] This fact is not completely explained by the increased

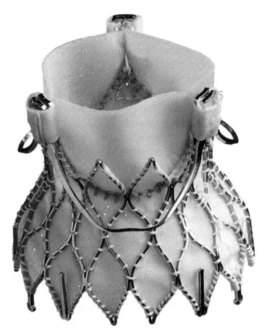

Fig. 4. Next-generation transcatheter heart valve III: Medtronic Engager aortic valve prosthesis for transapical use. (*Courtesy of* Medtronic, Minneapolis, MN; with permission.)

EuroSCORE for transapical patients compared with transfemoral patients. The periprocedural risk associated, for example, with peripheral arterial disease in patients without the transfemoral access option might not be ameliorated by choosing the transapical approach. However, these data emphasize the importance of optimal patient screening that should not be based on EuroSCORE evaluation alone.

A promising alternative for TAVI patients without transfemoral access options is the approach via the subclavian artery, which shows promising results.[14] In addition, the direct transaortic access, which is associated with a lower rate of vascular complications in TAVI patients, also provides direct control of the valve prosthesis during the procedure without the need for touching the heart itself (as with the transapical route).

STROKE RATE

Together with periprosthetic aortic regurgitation, the TAVI-associated stroke rate is a major issue of the procedure. In the PARTNER trial cohort A, the 30-day stroke rate was not significantly increased in TAVI patients compared with SAVR patients (3.8% vs 2.1%).[5] However, in up to 80% of all TAVI patients, silent cerebral embolism has been detected in recent MRI studies.[15]

Cerebral Protection Devices

Cerebral protection devices, which are temporarily introduced via transradial or transbrachial access into the supra-aortic arteries during the TAVI procedure, might help to reduce the TAVI-associated stroke rate. Two devices with different mechanisms (capture vs deflection of embolic material) have recently been used in experimental studies.

The Claret Tandem Embolic Protection Device (Claret Medical, Santa Rosa, CA, USA) consists of 2 filters that capture embolic material during the procedure (calcified parts of the native valve, thrombi, debris) and is introduced via transradial or transbrachial access over the right side of TAVI patients. A proximal filter is deployed in the innominate artery for the protection of the right vertebral artery and the right common carotid artery (**Fig. 5**A). Afterwards, the soft tip of the catheter may be advanced into the aortic arch and then deflected for an atraumatic intubation of the left common carotid artery with introduction of the distal filter (see **Fig. 5**B). After the TAVI procedure, calcified debris and/or thrombotic material is captured in the filters and removed from the body (see **Fig. 5**C and D).

The Embrella Embolic Deflector Device (Edwards Lifesciences, Irvine, CA, USA) is introduced via transradial or transbrachial access in TAVI patients. After introduction of the device through the innominate artery into the aortic arch, a self-expanding nitinol frame with a polyurethane membrane that does not interfere with cerebral perfusion is developed like an umbrella in the aortic arch (**Fig. 6**A)

and positioned in front of the origin of the supra-aortic vessels (see **Fig. 6**B). The embolic material is not captured in a filter, but is deflected into the peripheral circulation. This system caused no significant peripheral embolism in any patient in a recent feasibility study.[16]

Before widespread routine use of these devices can be recommended, cerebral protection devices have to show a significant reduction of the stroke rate in randomized controlled trials.

CONDUCTION DISTURBANCES

In the PARTNER trial cohort A, 5.7% of the TAVI patients suffered from conduction disturbances and were in need of a permanent pacemaker after the procedure. The permanent pacemaker implantation rate in this trial was not significantly different from that in SAVR patients. However, recent studies report a pacemaker rate of up to 40%, especially in patients who were treated with the Medtronic CoreValve system.[11,17]

TAVI Without Predilation

Balloon predilation of the stenosed aortic valve is currently thought to be a necessary step for valve preparation before device placement and is therefore considered to be an obligatory part of the procedure. Clear evidence supporting this policy is lacking. In contrast, predilation might be responsible

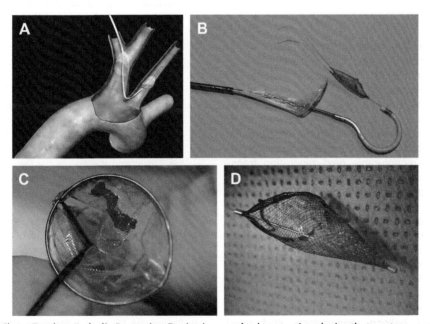

Fig. 5. The Claret Tandem Embolic Protection Device is a cerebral protection device that captures embolic material in 2 filters. The proximal filter is developed in the innominate artery, the distal filter in the left common carotid artery (*A, B*). Captured thromboembolic material in the proximal (*C*) and distal filter (*D*). (*Courtesy of Claret Medical, Santa Rosa, CA; with permission.*)

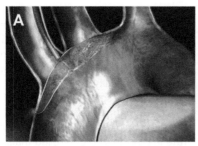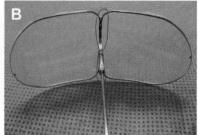

Fig. 6. The Embrella Embolic Deflector is a cerebral detection device that covers the origin of the supra-aortic vessels and deflects embolic material (*A*). This system, which consists of a nitinol frame with a polyurethane membrane (*B*), is introduced via transbrachial access over the innominate artery into the aortic arch. (*Courtesy of* Embrella/Edwards Lifesciences, Irvine, CA; with permission.)

for hemodynamic deterioration of patients with severely impaired left ventricular ejection fraction, embolization of thrombotic and valvular material, and might also be a major reason for postprocedural conduction disturbances.[18,19] A pilot study by Grube and colleagues[20] in 60 consecutive patients has recently shown that TAVI without balloon predilation is feasible and safe. Postdilation was necessary in only 17% of patients. The abandonment of balloon valvuloplasty in this study was associated with a significantly reduced permanent pacemaker rate compared with a historic control group (11.7% vs 27.8%) and showed comparable hemodynamic results without increase of the transvalvular gradient after the TAVI procedure.

SUMMARY

TAVI has been established as an alternative to SAVR in inoperable and high-risk patients with severe, symptomatic aortic stenosis. Several upcoming devices will optimize and facilitate the procedure to address these remaining TAVI-specific issues and to further reduce the rate of complications. Periprosthetic aortic regurgitation will be reduced by larger prosthesis sizes and re-positionable/recapturable next-generation trans-catheter heart valves. Upcoming sheaths and percutaneous closure devices will further reduce the rate of vascular complications and severe bleeding events. In patients without the possibility of transfemoral access, the trans-subclavian and the direct transaortic approaches have emerged as alternatives to the transapical approach. Cerebral protection devices might help to reduce the rate of strokes and especially the rate of clinically silent cerebral embolism in TAVI patients. Abandonment of balloon valvuloplasty and rapid ventricular pacing might not only facilitate the TAVI procedure but also improve outcome by reducing pacemaker and stroke rate. Thus,

younger and healthier individuals will also benefit from TAVI in the near future.

REFERENCES

1. Bonhoeffer P, Boudjemline Y, Saliba Z, et al. Percutaneous replacement of pulmonary valve in a right-ventricle to pulmonary-artery prosthetic conduit with valve dysfunction. Lancet 2000;356:1403–5.
2. Cribier A, Eltchaninoff H, Bash A, et al. Percutaneous transcatheter implantation of an aortic valve prosthesis for calcific aortic stenosis: first human case description. Circulation 2002;106:3006–8.
3. Grube E, Laborde JC, Gerckens U, et al. Percutaneous implantation of the CoreValve self-expanding valve prosthesis in high-risk patients with aortic valve disease: the Siegburg first-in-man study. Circulation 2006;114:1616–24.
4. Leon MB, Smith CR, Mack M, et al. Transcatheter aortic-valve implantation for aortic stenosis in patients who cannot undergo surgery. N Engl J Med 2010;363:1597–607.
5. Smith CR, Leon MB, Mack MJ, et al. Transcatheter versus surgical aortic-valve replacement in high-risk patients. N Engl J Med 2011;364:2187–98.
6. Sinning JM, Walenta K, Werner N, et al. Hotline update of clinical trials and registries presented at the 77th spring meeting of the German Society of Cardiology 2011. Clin Res Cardiol 2011;100(7):553–60.
7. Rallidis LS, Moyssakis IE, Ikonomidis I, et al. Natural history of early aortic paraprosthetic regurgitation: a five-year follow-up. Am Heart J 1999;138:351–7.
8. Abdel-Wahab M, Zahn R, Horack M, et al. Aortic regurgitation after transcatheter aortic valve implantation: incidence and early outcome. Results from the German transcatheter aortic valve interventions registry. Heart 2011;97:899–906.
9. Sinning JM, Ghanem A, Steinhauser H, et al. Renal function as predictor of mortality in patients after percutaneous transcatheter aortic valve implantation. JACC Cardiovasc Interv 2010;3:1141–9.

10. Tamburino C, Capodanno D, Ramondo A, et al. Incidence and predictors of early and late mortality after transcatheter aortic valve implantation in 663 patients with severe aortic stenosis. Circulation 2011;123:299–308.

11. Zahn R, Gerckens U, Grube E, et al. Transcatheter aortic valve implantation: first results from a multi-centre real-world registry. Eur Heart J 2011;32: 198–204.

12. Falk V, Walther T, Schwammenthal E, et al. Transapical aortic valve implantation with a self-expanding anatomically oriented valve. Eur Heart J 2011; 32(7):878–87.

13. Lefevre T, Kappetein AP, Wolner E, et al. One year follow-up of the multi-centre European PARTNER transcatheter heart valve study. Eur Heart J 2011; 32:148–57.

14. Petronio AS, De Carlo M, Bedogni F, et al. Safety and efficacy of the subclavian approach for transcatheter aortic valve implantation with the CoreValve revalving system. Circ Cardiovasc Interv 2010;3: 359–66.

15. Ghanem A, Muller A, Nahle CP, et al. Risk and fate of cerebral embolism after transfemoral aortic valve implantation a prospective pilot study with diffusion-weighted magnetic resonance imaging. J Am Coll Cardiol 2010;55:1427–32.

16. Schofer J, Bijuklic K, Webb JG, et al. First-in-man experience with a novel cerebral protection device for percutaneous aortic valve implantation. Presented at the 77th Spring Meeting of the German Society of Cardiology. Mannheim, April 29, 2011.

17. Rajani R, Kakad M, Khawaja MZ, et al. Paravalvular regurgitation one year after transcatheter aortic valve implantation. Catheter Cardiovasc Interv 2010;75:868–72.

18. Khawaja MZ, Rajani R, Cook A, et al. Permanent pacemaker insertion after CoreValve transcatheter aortic valve implantation: incidence and contributing factors (the UK CoreValve Collaborative). Circulation 2011;123:951–60.

19. Nuis RJ, Van Mieghem NM, Schultz CJ, et al. Timing and potential mechanisms of new conduction abnormalities during the implantation of the Medtronic CoreValve System in patients with aortic stenosis. Eur Heart J 2011;32(16):2067–74.

20. Grube E, Naber C, Abizaid A, et al. Feasibility of transcatheter aortic valve implantation without balloon predilation: a pilot study. JACC Cardiovasc Interv 2011;4:751–5.

Percutaneous Mitral Balloon Valvuloplasty for Patients with Rheumatic Mitral Stenosis

Igor F. Palacios, MD[a,b,*], Dabit Arzamendi, MD, MSc[a]

KEYWORDS

- Percutaneous mitral balloon valvuloplasty • Mitral stenosis
- Heart disease lesions • Surgical mitral commissurotomy

Before 1982 cardiac surgery was the conventional form of treatment of symptomatic stenotic valvular heart disease lesions. Today, percutaneous balloon dilatation of stenotic cardiac valves is used in many centers for the treatment of patients with pulmonic, mitral, aortic, and tricuspid stenosis. Since its introduction in 1984 by Inoue and colleagues,[1–11] percutaneous mitral balloon valvuloplasty (PMV) has been used successfully as an alternative to open or closed surgical mitral commissurotomy in the treatment of patients with symptomatic rheumatic mitral stenosis.[12–35] PMV produces good immediate hemodynamic outcome, low complication rates, and clinical improvement in the majority of patients with mitral stenosis. PMV is safe and effective and provides sustained clinical and hemodynamic improvement in patients with rheumatic mitral stenosis. The immediate and long-term results seem similar to those of surgical mitral commissurotomy.[12–35] Today, PMV is the preferred form of therapy for relief of mitral stenosis for a selected group of patients with symptomatic mitral stenosis.

PATIENT SELECTION

Selection of patients for PMV should be based on symptoms, physical examination, and 2-D and Doppler echocardiographic findings.[4,17] PMV is usually performed electively. Emergency PMV can be performed, however, as a life-saving procedure in patients with mitral stenosis and severe pulmonary edema refractory to medical therapy and/or cardiogenic shock. Patients considered for PMV should be symptomatic (New York Heart Association [NYHA] $\geq$ class II), should have no recent thromboembolic events, have less than 2 grades of mitral regurgitation (MR) by contrast ventriculography (using the Sellers classification[36]), and have no evidence of left atrial thrombus on 2-D and transesophageal echocardiography (**Table 1**). Transthoracic and transesophageal echocardiography should be performed routinely before PMV. Patients in atrial fibrillation and patients with previous embolic episodes should be anticoagulated with warfarin with a therapeutic prothrombin time for at least 3 months before PMV. Patients with left atrium thrombus on 2-D echocardiography should be excluded. PMV could be performed, however, in these patients if left atrium thrombus has resolved after warfarin therapy.

PMV success depends on appropriate patient selection. A multifactorial score derived from clinical, anatomic/echocardiographic, and hemodynamic variables predicts procedural success and clinical outcome (**Fig. 1**).[25] Demographic data, echocardiographic parameters (including

Adapted from Palacios IF. Percutaneous mitral balloon valvuloplasty for patients with rheumatic mitral stenosis. In Herrmann HC, ed. Interventional Cardiology: Percutaneous Noncoronary Intervention. Totowa, NJ: Humana Press; 2005:3–27; with kind permission from Springer Science+Business Media.

[a] Heart Center, Massachusetts General Hospital, Boston, MA 02114, USA
[b] Harvard Medical School, Boston, MA, USA
* Corresponding author. Heart Center, Massachusetts General Hospital, Boston, MA 02114.
E-mail address: ipalacios@partners.org

Table 1
Recommendations for percutaneous mitral valvuloplasty

Current Indication	Class	Level of Evidence
Symptomatic patients (NYHA functional class II, III, or IV), moderate or severe mitral stenosis (area <1.5 cm^2), and valve morphology favorable for percutaneous balloon valvuloplasty in the absence of left atrial thrombus or moderate to severe MR	I	Grade A
Asymptomatic patients with moderate or severe mitral stenosis (area <1.5 cm^2) and valve morphology favorable for percutaneous balloon valvuloplasty who have pulmonary hypertension (pulmonary artery systolic pressure >50 mm Hg at rest or 60 mm Hg with exercise) in the absence of left atrial thrombus or moderate to severe MR	IIa	Grade C
Patients with NYHA functional class III–IV, moderate or severe mitral stenosis (area <1.5 cm^2), and a nonpliable calcified valve who are at high risk for surgery in the absence of left atrial thrombus or moderate to severe MR	IIa	Grade B
Asymptomatic patients, moderate or severe mitral stenosis (area <1.5 cm^2), and valve morphology favorable for percutaneous balloon valvuloplasty who have new onset of atrial fibrillation in the absence of left atrial thrombus or moderate to severe MR	IIb	Grade B
Patients in NYHA functional class III–IV, moderate or severe mitral stenosis (area <1.5 cm^2), and a nonpliable calcified valve who are low-risk candidates for surgery	IIb	Grade C
Patients with mild mitral stenosis	III	Grade C

Adapted from current American College of Cardiology/American Heart Association and European guidelines for the management of patients with valvular heart disease.

echocardiographic score [**Fig. 2**]), and procedure-related variables recorded from 1085 consecutive patients who underwent PMV at Massachusetts General Hospital, and their long-term clinical follow-up (death, mitral valve replacement, and redo PMV) were used to derive this clinical score. Multivariate regression analysis of the first 800 procedures was performed to identify independent predictors of procedural success. Significant variables were formulated into a risk score and validated prospectively. Six independent predictors

of PMV success were identified: age less than 55 years, NYHA classes I and II, pre-PMV mitral area of 1 cm^2 or greater, pre-PMV MR grade less than 2, echocardiographic score of 8 or greater, and male gender.[17,36] A score was constructed from the arithmetic sum of variables present per patient. Procedural success rates increased incrementally with increasing score (0% for 0/6, 39.7% for 1/6, 54.4% for 2/6, 77.3% for 3/6, 85.7% for 4/6, 95% for 5/6, and 100% for 6/6; P<.001). In a validation cohort (n = 285 procedures), the multifactorial score remained a significant predictor of PMV success (P<.001). Comparison between the new score and the echocardiographic score confirmed that the new index was more sensitive and specific (P<.001). This new score also predicts long-term outcomes (P<.001). Clinical, anatomic, and hemodynamic variables predict PMV success and clinical outcome and may be formulated in a scoring system that would help to identify the best candidates for PMV.[25]

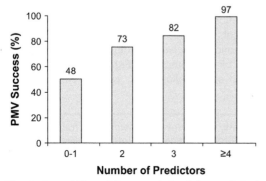

Fig. 1. A multifactorial score derived from clinical, anatomic/echocardiographic, and hemodynamic variables would predict procedural success and clinical outcome.

TECHNIQUE OF PMV

PMV is performed with patients in the fasting state under mild sedation. Antibiotics (dicloxacillin, 500 mg by mouth every 6 hours for 4 doses started before the procedure, or cefazolin, 1 g intravenous

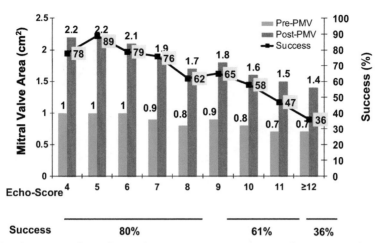

Fig. 2. Relationship between echocardiographic score, pre-PMV MVA, and post-PMV MVA, and immediate success after PMV. (*From* Palacios IF. Percutaneous mitral balloon valvuloplasty for patients with rheumatic mitral stenosis. In Herrmann HC, ed. Interventional Cardiology: Percutaneous Noncoronary Intervention. Totowa, NJ: Humana Press; 2005:3–27; with permission.)

[IV] at the time of the procedure) are used. Patients allergic to penicillin should receive vancomycin (1 g IV) at the time of the procedure.

All patients carefully chosen as candidates for mitral balloon valvuloplasty should undergo diagnostic right and left and transseptal left heart catheterization. After transseptal left heart catheterization, systemic anticoagulation is achieved by the intravenous administration of 100 U/kg of heparin. In patients older than 40 years, coronary arteriogaphy is recommended and should also be performed.

Hemodynamic measurements, cardiac output, and cine left ventriculography are performed before and after PMV. Cardiac output is measured by thermodilution and Fick method techniques. Mitral valve calcification and angiographic severity of MR (Sellers classification) are graded qualitatively from 0 grade to 4 grades.[36] An oxygen diagnostic run is performed before and after PMV to determine the presence of left-to-right shunt across the atrial septum after PMV.

There is not a unique technique for PMV. Most of the techniques for PMV require transseptal left heart catheterization and use of the antegrade approach.[4,12–22,24–28] Antegrade PMV can be accomplished using a single-balloon (**Fig. 3**B) or a double-balloon technique (see **Fig. 3**A). In this latter approach, the two balloons could be placed through a single femoral vein and single transseptal punctures or through two femoral veins and two separate atrial septal punctures. In the retrograde technique of PMV, the balloon dilating catheters are advanced percutaneously through the right and left femoral arteries over guide wires that have been snared from the descending aorta. These guide wires have been advanced transseptaly from

the right femoral vein into the left atrium, the left ventricle, and the ascending aorta.[26] A retrograde nontransseptal technique of PMV has also been described.[12] Recently, a technique of PMV using a newly designed metallic valvulotome was introduced.[13] The device consists of a detachable metallic cylinder with 2 articulated bars screwed onto the distal end of a disposable catheter whose proximal end is connected to activating pliers. Squeezing the pliers opens the bars up to a maximum of 40 mm (see **Fig. 3**C). The results with this device are at least comparable to those of the other balloon techniques of PMV.[13] Multiple uses after sterilization, however, should markedly decrease procedural costs.

The Antegrade Double-Balloon Technique

In performing PMV using the antegrade double-balloon technique (see **Fig. 3**), two 0.0038-in, 260-cm long polytetrafluorethylene (Teflon)-coated exchange wires are placed across the mitral valve into the left ventricle, through the aortic valve into the ascending and then the descending aorta.[4–17] Care should be taken to maintain large and smooth loops of the guide wires in the left ventricular cavity to allow appropriate placement of the dilating balloons. If a second guide wire cannot be placed into the ascending and descending aorta, a 0.038-in Amplatz-type transfer guide wire with a preformed curlew at its tip can be placed at the left ventricular apex. In patients with an aortic valve prosthesis, both guide wires with performed curlew tips should be placed at the left ventricular apex. When one or both guide wires are placed in the left ventricular apex, the balloons should be inflated sequentially. Care should be taken to avoid forward

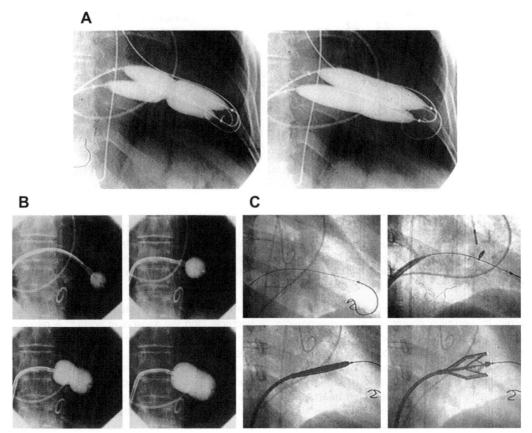

Fig. 3. Different percutaneous approaches of PMV: the double-balloon technique (*A*), the Inoue technique (*B*), and the metallic valvulotome (*C*). (*From* Palacios IF. Percutaneous mitral balloon valvuloplasty for patients with rheumatic mitral stenosis. In Herrmann HC, ed. Interventional Cardiology: Percutaneous Noncoronary Intervention. Totowa, NJ: Humana Press; 2005:3–27; with permission.)

movement of the balloons and guide wires to prevent left ventricular perforation. Two balloon dilatation catheters, chosen according to patient body surface area (BSA), are then advanced over each one of the guide wires and positioned across the mitral valve parallel to the longitudinal axis of the left ventricle. The balloon valvotomy catheters are then inflated by hand until the indentation produced by the stenotic mitral valve is no longer seen. Generally one, but occasionally two or three, inflations are performed. After complete deflation, the balloons are removed sequentially.

The Inoue Technique of PMV

PMV can also been performed using the Inoue technique (see **Fig. 3**B).[1,8,15] The Inoue balloon is a 12-French shaft, coaxial, double-lumen catheter. The balloon is made of a double layer of rubber tubing with a layer of synthetic micromesh in between. After transseptal catheterization, a stainless steel guide wire is advanced through the transspetal catheter and placed with its tip coiled into the left atrium and the transseptal

catheter removed. A 14-French dilator is advanced over the guide wire and used to dilate the femoral vein and the atrial septum. A balloon catheter chosen according to patient height is advanced over the guide wire into the left atrium. The distal part of the balloon is inflated and advanced into the left ventricle with the help of the spring wire stylet, which has been inserted through the inner lumen of the catheter. Once the catheter is in the left ventricle, the partially inflated balloon is moved back and forth inside the left ventricle to assure that it is free of the chordae tendinae. The catheter is then gently pulled against the mitral plane until resistance is felt. The balloon is then rapidly inflated to its full capacity and then deflated quickly. During inflation of the balloon, an indentation should be seen in its midportion. The catheter is withdrawn into the left atrium and the mitral gradient and cardiac output measured. If further dilatations are required, the stylet is introduced again and the sequence of steps (described previously) repeated at a larger balloon volume. After each dilatation, its effect should be assessed by pressure measurement, auscultation, and 2-D echocardiography. If MR occurs, further dilation of the valve should not be performed.

MECHANISM OF PMV

The mechanism of successful PMV is splitting of the fused commissures toward the mitral annulus, resulting in commissural widening. This mechanism has been demonstrated by pathologic, surgical, and echocardiographic studies.[28–31] In addition, in patients with calcific mitral stenosis, the balloons could increase mitral valve flexibility by the fracture of the calcified deposits in the mitral valve leaflets.[28] Although rare, undesirable complications, such as leaflets tears, left ventricular perforation, tear of the atrial septum, and rupture of chordae, mitral annulus, and papillary muscle, could also occur.

IMMEDIATE OUTCOME

Fig. 3 shows the hemodynamic changes produced by PMV in one patient. PMV resulted in a significant decrease in mitral gradient, mean left atrium pressure, and mean pulmonary artery pressure and an increase in cardiac output and mitral valve area (MVA). **Table 2** shows the changes in MVA reported by several investigators using different techniques of PMV. In most series, PMV is reported to increase MVA from less than 1.0 cm^2 to approximately 2.0 cm^2.[2–27,32,34–37,39,40]

At Massachusetts General Hospital, between July 1986 and July 2000, 879 consecutive patients with mitral stenosis underwent 939 PMVs.[17] As shown in **Fig. 4**, in this group of patients, PMV

resulted in a significant decrease in mitral gradient from 14 ± 6 to 6 ± 3 mm Hg. The mean cardiac output significantly increased from 3.9 ± 1.1 to 4.5 ± 1.3 L/min and the calculated MVA from 0.9 ± 0.3 to 1.9 ± 0.7 cm^2. In addition, mean pulmonary artery pressure significantly decreased from 36 ± 13 to 29 ± 11 mm Hg and the mean left atrial pressure decreased from 25 ± 7 to 17 ± 7 mm Hg and, consequently, the calculated pulmonary vascular resistances decreased significantly after PMV.[17]

A successful hemodynamic outcome (defined as a post-PMV MVA ≥1.5 cm^2 and post-PMV MR <3 Sellers grade) was obtained in 72% of the patients. Although a suboptimal result occurred in 28% of the patients, a post-PMV MVA less than or equal to 1.0 cm^2 (critical MVA) was present in only 8.7% of these patients.

PREDICTORS OF INCREASE IN MITRAL VALVE AREA AND PROCEDURAL SUCCESS WITH PMV

Univariate analysis demonstrated that the increase in MVA with PMV is directly related to the balloon size used because it reflects in the effective balloon dilating area (EBDA) and is inversely related to the echocardiographic score (see **Fig. 2**), the presence of atrial fibrillation, the presence of fluoroscopic calcium, the presence of previous surgical commissurotomy, older age, NYHA pre-PMV, and presence of MR before PMV. Multiple stepwise regression analysis identified balloon size ($P<.02$), the echocardiographic score ($P<.0001$), and the presence of atrial fibrillation ($P<.009$) and MR before PMV ($P<.03$) as independent predictors of the increase in MVA with PMV.[17]

Table 2
Immediate changes in mitral valve area after percutaneous mitral valvuloplasty

Author	Institution	No. Patients	Age	Pre-PMV	Post-PMV
Palacios et al[17]	MGH	879	55 ± 15	0.9 ± 0.3	1.9 ± 0.7
Vahanian[45]	Tenon	1024	45 ± 15	1.0 ± 0.2	1.9 ± 0.3
Hernández et al[14]	Clínico Madrid	561	53 ± 13	1.0 ± 0.2	1.8 ± 0.4
Stefanadis et al[12]	Athens University	438	44 ± 11	1.0 ± 0.3	2.1 ± 0.5
Chen et al[8]	Guangzhou	4832	37 ± 12	1.1 ± 0.3	2.1 ± 0.2
NHLBI[9]	Multicenter	738	54 ± 12	1.0 ± 0.4	2.0 ± 0.2
Inoue et al[1]	Takeda	527	50 ± 10	1.1 ± 0.1	2.0 ± 0.1
Inoue registry[62]	Multicenter	1251	53 ± 15	1.0 ± 0.3	1.8 ± 0.6
Ben Farhat et al[23]	Fattouma	463	33 ± 12	1.0 ± 0.2	2.2 ± 0.4
Arora et al[20]	G.B. Pan	600	27 ± 8	0.8 ± 0.2	2.2 ± 0.4
Cribier et al[13]	Rouen	153	36 ± 15	1.0 ± 0.2	2.2 ± 0.4

Abbreviations: MGH, Massachusetts General Hospital; NHLBI, National Heart, Lung, and Blood Institute.
Data from Palacios IF. Percutaneous mitral balloon valvuloplasty for patients with rheumatic mitral stenosis. In Herrmann HC, ed. Interventional Cardiology: Percutaneous Noncoronary Intervention. Totowa, NJ: Humana Press; 2005:3–27.

Immediate Outcome

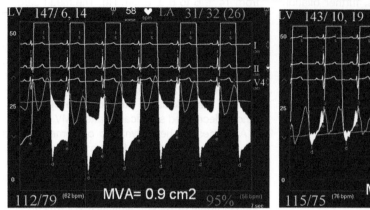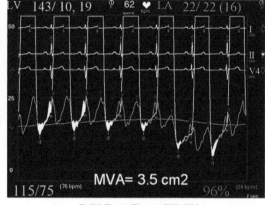

LV/LA Pre-PMV   LV/LA Post-PMV

Fig. 4. Hemodynamic changes produced by a successful PMV in one patient with severe mitral stenosis. Simultaneous left atrium (LA) and left ventricular (LV) pressures before (*left*) and after (*right*) PMV. The corresponding calculated MVAs are also displayed. (*From* Palacios IF. Percutaneous mitral balloon valvuloplasty for patients with rheumatic mitral stenosis. In Herrmann HC, ed. Interventional Cardiology: Percutaneous Noncoronary Intervention. Totowa, NJ: Humana Press; 2005:3–27; with permission.)

Univariate predictors of procedural success included age, pre-PMV MVA, mean pre-PMV pulmonary artery pressure, male gender, echocardiographic score, pre-PMV MR greater than or equal to 2+, history of previous surgical commissurotomy, presence of atrial fibrillation, and presence of mitral valve calcification under fluoroscopy.[17]

Multiple stepwise logistic regression analysis identified larger pre-PMV MVA (odds ratio [OR] 13.05; 95% CI, 7.74 to 22.51; P<.001), less degree of pre-PMV MR (OR 3.85; 95% CI, 2.27 to 6.66; P<.001), younger age (OR 3.33; 95% CI, 1.41 to 7.69; P = .006), absence of previous surgical commissurotomy (OR 1.85; 95% CI, 1.20 to 2.86; P = .004), male gender (OR 1.92; 95% CI, 1.19 to 3.13; P = .008), and echocardiographic score less than or equal to 8 (OR 1.69; 95% CI, 1.18 to 2.44; P = .004).

The Echocardiographic Score

The echocardiographic examination of the mitral valve can acccurately characterize the severity and extent of the pathologic process in patients with mitral stenosis. The most used score to identify the anatomic abnormalities of the stenotic mitral valve is that described by Wilkins and colleagues[31] (see **Fig. 2**; **Table 3**). This echocardiographic score is an important predictor of the immediate and long-term outcome of PMV. In this morphologic score, each of the following—leaflet rigidity, leaflet thickening, valvular calcification, and subvalvular disease—is scored from 0 to 4. A higher score represents a heavily calcified, thickened, and immobile valve with extensive thickening

and calcification of the subvalvular apparatus. The increase in MVA with PMV is inversely related to the echocardiographic score. The best outcome with PMV occurs in those patients with echocardiographic scores less than or equal to 8. The increase in MVA is significantly greater in patients with echocardiographic scores less than or equal to 8 than in those with echocardiographic score greater than 8. Among the 4 components of the echocardiographic score, valve leaflets thickening and subvalvular disease correlate the best with the increase in MVA produced by PMV.[31–33] Therefore, suboptimal results with PMV are more likely to occur in patients with valves that are more rigid and more thickened and in those with more subvalvular fibrosis and calcification.

Balloon Size and EBDA

The increase in MVA with PMV is directly related to balloon size. This effect was first demonstrated in a subgroup of patients who underwent repeat PMV.[34] They initially underwent PMV with a single balloon resulting in a mean MVA of 1.2 ± 0.2 cm². They underwent repeat PMV using the double-balloon technique, which increased the EBDA normalized by BSA (EBDA/BSA) from 3.41 ± 0.2 to 4.51 ± 0.2 cm²/m². The mean MVA in this group after repeat PMV was 1.8 cm² ± 0.7 cm². The increase in MVA in patients who underwent PMV at Massachusetts General Hospital using the double-balloon technique (EBDA of 6.4 ± 0.03 cm²) was significantly greater than the increase in MVA achieved in patients who underwent PMV using the single-balloon technique (EBDA of 4.3

Table 3
Echocardiographic score

Grade	Leaflet Mobility	Valvular Thickening	Valvular Calcification	Subvalvular Thickening
0	Normal	Normal	Normal	Normal
1	Highly mobile valve with restriction of only the leaflet tips	Leaflet near normal (4–5 mm)	A single area of increased echo brightness	Minimal thickening of chordal structures just below the valve
2	Middle portion and base of leaflets have reduced mobility	Midleaflet thickening, marked thickening of the margins	Scattered areas of brightness confined to leaflet margins	Thickening of chordae extending up to one-third of chordal length
3	Valve leaflets move forward in diastole mainly at the base	Thickening extending through the entire leaflets (5–8 mm)	Brightness extending into the midportion of leaflets	Thickening extending to the distal third of the chordae
4	No or minimal forward movement of the leaflets in diastole	Marked thickening of all leaflet tissue (>8–10 mm)	Extensive brightness throughout most of the leaflet tissue	Extensive thickening and shortening of all chordae extending down to the papillary muscles

Echocardiographic grading of the severity and extent of the anatomic abnormalities in patients with mitral stenosis. The total score is the sum of each of these echocardiographic features (maximum 16).

$\pm$ 0.02 cm^2). The mean MVAs were 1.9 $\pm$ 0.7 and 1.4 $\pm$ 0.1 cm^2 for patients who underwent PMV with the double-balloon and the single-balloon techniques, respectively. However, care should be taken in the selection of dilating balloon catheters so as to obtain an adequate final MVA and no change or a minimal increase in MR.

Mitral Valve Calcification

The immediate outcome of patients undergoing PMV is inversely related to the severity of valvular calcification seen by fluoroscopy. Patients without fluoroscopic calcium have a greater increase in MVA after PMV than patients with calcified valves. Patients with either no or 1+ fluoroscopic calcium have a greater increase in MVA after PMV (1.1 $\pm$ 0.6 cm^2 and 0.9 $\pm$ 0.5 cm^2, respectively) than those patients with 2, 3, or 4 + of calcium (0.8 $\pm$ 0.6, 0.8 $\pm$ 0.5, and 0.6 $\pm$ 0.4 cm^2, respectively).[42]

Previous Surgical Commissurotomy

Although the increase in MVA with PMV is inversely related to the presence of previous surgical mitral commissurotomy, PMV can produce a good outcome in this group of patients. The post-PMV mean MVA in 154 patients with previous surgical commissurotomy was 1.8 $\pm$ 0.7 cm^2 compared with a valve area of 1.9 $\pm$ 0.6 cm^2 in patients without previous surgical commissurotomy ($P<.05$). In this group of patients, an echocardiographic score less than or equal to 8 was an important predictor of a successful hemodynamic immediate outcome.[43–46]

Age

The immediate outcome of PMV is directly related to the age of the patient. The percentage of patients obtaining a good result with this technique decreases as age increases. A successful hemodynamic outcome from PMV was obtained in fewer than 50% of patients age 65 years or older.[34] This inverse relationship between age and the immediate outcome from PMV is due to the higher frequency of atrial fibrillation, calcified valves, and higher echocardiographic scores in elderly patients.[34,35]

Atrial Fibrillation

The increase in MVA with PMV is inversely related to the presence of atrial fibrillation; the post-PMV MVA of patients in normal sinus rhythm was 2.0 ± 0.7 cm^2 compared with a valve area of 1.7 ± 0.6 cm^2 of those patients in atrial fibrillation.[47] The inferior immediate outcome of PMV in patients with mitral stenosis who are in atrial fibrillation is more likely related to the presence of clinical and morphologic characteristics associated with inferior results after PMV. Patients in atrial fibrillation are older and present more frequently with echocardiographic scores greater than 8, NYHA functional class IV, calcified mitral valves under fluoroscopy, and a previous history of surgical mitral commissurotomy.[47]

Mitral Regurgitation Before PMV

The presence and severity of MR before PMV is an independent predictor of unfavorable outcome of PMV. The increase in mitral valve after PMV is inversely related to the severity of MR determined by angiography before the procedure. This inverse relationship between presence of MR and immediate outcome of PMV is in part due to the higher frequency of atrial fibrillation, higher echocardiographic scores, calcified mitral valves under fluoroscopy, and older age in patients with MR before PMV.

COMPLICATIONS

Table 4 shows the complications reported by several investigators after PMV.[1–27,32,34–37,39,40] Mortality and morbidity with PMV are low and similar to surgical commissurotomy. Overall, there is less than 1% mortality. Severe MR (4 grades by angiography) has been reported in 1% to 5.2% of the patients. Some of these patients required in-hospital mitral valve replacement. Thromboembolic episodes and stroke has been reported in 0 to 3.1% and pericardial tamponade in 0.2% to 4.6% of cases in these series. Pericardial tamponade can occur from transseptal catheterization and more rarely from ventricular perforation. PMV is associated with a 3% to 16% incidence of left-to-right shunt immediately after the procedure. The the pulmonary-to-systemic flow ratio (QP/QS), however, is greater than or equal to 2:1 in only a minimum number of patients.

The authors have demonstrated that severe MR (4 grades by angiography) occurs in approximately 3% of patients undergoing PMV.[37] An undesirable increase in MR (≥2 grades by angiography) occurred in 10.1% of patients. This undesirable increase in MR is well tolerated in most patients. Furthermore, more than half of them have less MR at follow-up cardiac catheterization. The authors have demonstrated that the EBDA/BSA ratio is the only predictor of increased MR after PMV.[37] The EBDA is calculated using standard geometric formulas. The incidence of MR is lower if balloon sizes are chosen so that EBDA/BSA is less than or equal to 4.0 cm^2/m^2. The single-balloon technique results in a lower incidence of MR but provides less relief of mitral stenosis than the double-balloon technique. Thus, there is an optimal EBDA between 3.1 and 4.0 cm^2/m^2, which achieves a maximal MVA with a minimal increase in MR. An echocardiographic score for the mitral valve that can predict the development of severe MR after PMV has also been described.[32] This score takes into account the distribution (even or

Table 4
Complications after percutaneous mitral valvuloplasty

Author	No. patients	Mortality	Tamponade	Severe MR	Embolism
Palacios et al[17]	879	0.6%	1.0%	3.4%	1.8%
Vahanian[45]	1024	0.4%	0.3%	3.4%	0.3%
Hernández et al[14]	561	0.4%	0.6%	4.5%	
Stefanadis et al[12]	438	0.2%	0.0%	3.4%	0.0%
Chen et al[8]	4832	0.1%	0.8%	1.4%	0.5%
NHLBI[9]	738	3.0%	4.0%	3.0%	3.0%
Inoue et al[1]	527	0.0%	1.6%	1.9%	0.6%
Inoue registry[62]	1251	0.6%	1.4%	3.8%	0.9%
Ben Farhat et al[23]	463	0.4%	0.7%	4.6%	2.0%
Arora et al[20]	600	1.0%	1.3%	1.0%	0.5%
Cribier et al[13]	153	0.0%	0.7%	1.4%	0.7%

Abbreviation: NHLBI, National Heart, Lung, and Blood Institute.

uneven) of leaflet thickening and calcification, the degree and symmetry of commissural disease, and the severity of subvalvular disease.

Left-to-right shunt through the created atrial communication occurred in 3% to 16% of the patients undergoing PMV. The size of the defect is small as reflected in a QP/QS of less than 2:1 in the majority of patients. Older age, fluoroscopic evidence of mitral valve calcification, higher echocardiographic score, pre-PMV lower cardiac output, and higher pre-PMV NYHA functional class are the factors that predispose patients to develop left-to-right shunt post-PMV.[38] Clinical, echocardiographic, surgical, and hemodynamic follow-up of patients with post-PMV left-to-right shunt demonstrated that the defect closed in approximately 60%. Persistent left-to-right shunt at follow-up is small (QP/QS <2:1) and clinically well tolerated. In the series from Massachusetts General Hospital, there is one patient in whom the atrial shunt remained hemodynamically significant at follow-up. This patient underwent percutaneous transcatheter closure of her atrial defect with a clamshell device. Desideri and colleagues[40] reported atrial shunting determined by color flow transthoracic echocardiography in 61% of 57 patients immediately after PMV. The shunt persisted in 30% of patients at 19 ± 6 (range 9–33) months' follow-up. They identified the magnitude of the post-PMV atrial shunt (QP/QS >1.5:1), use of bifoil balloon (2 balloons on 1 shaft), and smaller post-PMV MVA as independent predictors of the persistence of atrial shunt at long-term follow-up.

CLINICAL FOLLOW-UP

Long-term follow-up studies after PMV are encouraging.[2–27,33–35] After PMV, the majority of patients have marked clinical improvement and become NYHA class I or II. The symptomatic, echocardiographic, and hemodynamic improvement produced by PMV persists in intermediate and long-term follow-up. The best long-term results are seen in patients with echocardiographic scores

less than or equal to 8. When PMV produces a good immediate outcome in this group of patients, restenosis is unlikely to occur at follow-up. Although PMV can result in a good outcome in patients with echocardiographic scores greater than 8, hemodynamic and echocardiographic restenosis is frequently demonstrated at follow-up despite ongoing clinical improvement. **Table 5** shows long-term follow-up results of patients undergoing PMV at different institutes. The authors reported an estimated 12-year survival rate of 74% in a cohort of 879 patients undergoing PMV at Massachusetts General Hospital (**Fig. 5**). Death at follow-up was directly related to age, post-PMV pulmonary artery pressure, and pre-PMV NYHA functional class IV. In the same group of patients, the 12-year event-free survival (alive and free of mitral valve replacement or repair and redo PMV) was 33% (**Fig. 6**). Cox regression analysis identified age (risk ratio[RR] 1.02; 95% CI, 1.01–1.03; $P<.0001$), pre-PMV NYHA functional class IV (RR 1.35; 95% CI, 1.00–1.81; $P = .05$), prior commissurotomy (RR .150; 95% CI, 1.16–1.92; $P = .002$), the echocardiographic score (RR 1.31; 95% CI, 1.02–1.67; $P = .003$), pre-PMV MR greater than or equal to 2+ (RR 1.56; 95% CI, 1.09–2.22; $P = .02$), post-PMV MR greater than or equal to 3+ (RR 3.54; 95% CI, 2.61–4.72; $P<.0001$), and post-PMV mean pulmonary artery pressure (RR 1.02; 95% CI, 1.01–1.03; $P<.0001$) as independent predictors of combined events at long-term follow-up.[17]

Actuarial survival and event-free survival rates throughout the follow-up period were significantly better in patients with echocardiographic scores less than or equal to 8. Survival rates were 82% for patients with echocardiographic score less than or equal to 8 and 57% for patients with score greater than 8 at a follow-up time of 12 years ($P<.0001$). Event-free survival (38% vs 22%; $P<.0001$) at 12 years' follow-up was also significantly higher for patients with echocardiographic score less than or equal to 8. Similar follow-up studies have been reported in other series with

Table 5
Clinical long-term follow-up after percutaneous mitral valvuloplasty

Author	No. Patients	Age	Follow-Up (years)	Survival	Event-Free Survival
Palacios et al[17]	879	55	12	74%	33%
Iung et al[15]	1024	49	10	85%	56%
Hernández et al[14]	561	53	7	95%	69%
Orrange et al[10]	132	44	7	83%	65%
Ben Farhat et al[23]	30	29	7	100%	90%
Stefanadis et al[12]	441	44	9	98%	75%

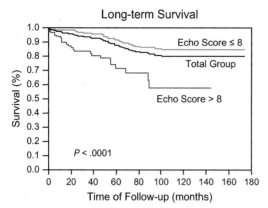

Fig. 5. Fifteen-year survival for all patients and for patients with echocardiographic score ≤8 and >8 undergoing PMV at Massachusetts General Hospital.

the double-balloon technique and with the Inoue technique of PMV.[21,23,40] More than 90% of young patients with pliable valves, in sinus rhythm and with no evidence of calcium under fluoroscopy, remain free of cardiovascular events at an approximately follow-up of 5 years.[21,23,40]

Functional deterioration at follow-up is late and related primarily to mitral restenosis.[23,40] The incidence of restenosis, as assessed by sequential echocardiography, is approximately 40% after 7 years.[25] Repeat PMV can be proposed if recurrent stenosis leads to symptoms. Currently, there are only a few series available on redo PMV. They show encouraging results in selected patients with favorable characteristics when restenosis

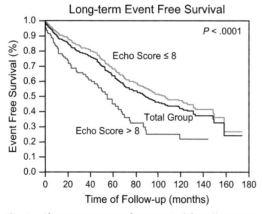

Fig. 6. Fifteen-year event-free survival for all patients and for patients with echocardiographic score ≤8 and >8 undergoing PMV at Massachusetts General Hospital. (*Data from* Palacios IF, Sanchez PL, Harrell LC, Weyman AE, Block PC. Which patients benefit from percutaneous mitral balloon valvuloplasty? Prevalvuloplasty and postvalvuloplasty variables that predict long-term outcome. Circulation 2002;105:1465–71.)

occurs several years after an initially successful procedure and if the predominant mechanism of restenosis is commissural refusion.[45]

Follow-Up in the Elderly

Tuzcu and colleagues[35] reported the outcome of PMV in 99 elderly patients (65 years or older). A successful outcome (valve area ≥1.5 cm² without ≥2+ increase in MR and without left-to-right shunt of ≥1.5: 1) was achieved in 46 patients. The best multivariate predictor of success was the combination of echocardiographic score, NYHA functional class, and inverse of MVA. Patients who had an unsuccessful outcome from PMV were in a higher NYHA functional class and had higher echocardiographic scores and smaller MVAs pre-PMV compared with those patients who had a successful outcome. Actuarial survival and combined event-free survival at 3 years were significantly better in the successful group. Mean follow-up was 16 ± 1 months. Actuarial survival (79 ± 7% vs 62 ± 10%; P = .04), survival without mitral valve replacement (71 ± 8% vs 41 ± 8%; P = .002), and event-free survival (54 ± 12% vs 38 ± 8%; P = .01) at 3 years were significantly better in the successful group of 46 patients than the unsuccessful group of 53 patients. Low echocardiographic score was the independent predictor of survival and lack of mitral valve calcification was the strongest predictor of event-free survival.

Data reported from 96 patients 75 and older have shown that these patients present a lower pre-PMV MVA (0.8 ± 0.3 vs 0.9 ± 0.3; P = .005), a lower post-PMV MVA (1.6 ± 0.6 vs 1.9 ± 0.7; P<.0001), and a lower procedural success (51.0% vs 71.4%; P<.0001) compared with patients younger than 75 years.[51] Patients 75 and older exhibited higher in-hospital mortality than patients younger than 75 (3.1% vs 0.3%) with no significant differences in the other procedure-related complications (cardiac tamponade, severe MR, significant left-to-right shunt, and embolism). Although in-hospital mortality was higher, in the majority of these patients PMV was considered a palliative treatment. Technical complications were similar, however, to those more favorable patients, ages younger than 75. Survival and event-free survival rates were 60% and 49% for patients 75 years and older at a follow-up time of 3 years. The echocardiographic score is an imperfect predictor of hemodynamic improvement in elderly patients.[17,25,35,36]

Unfortunately, no randomized study is available for elderly patients and a comparison of the results of PMV with those of surgical series is difficult because of the differences in the patients and surgical techniques involved.

Follow-Up of Patients with Calcified Mitral Valves

The presence of fluoroscopically visible calcification on the mitral valve influences the success of PMV. Patients with heavily ($\geq$3 grades) calcified valves under fluoroscopy have a poorer immediate outcome as reflected in a smaller post-PMV MVA and greater post-PMV mitral valve gradient. Immediate outcome is progressively worse as the calcification becomes more severe. The long-term results of PMV are significantly different in calcified and uncalcified groups and in subgroups of the calcified group.[42] The estimated 2-year survival is significantly lower for patients with calcified mitral valves than for those with uncalcified valves (80% vs 99%). The survival curve becomes worse as the severity of valvular calcification becomes more severe. Freedom from mitral valve replacement at 2 years was significantly lower for patients with calcified valves than for those with uncalcified valves (67% vs 93%). Similarly, the estimated event-free survival at 2 years in the calcified group became significantly poorer as the severity of calcification increased. The estimated event-free survival at 2 years was significantly lower for the calcified than for the uncalcified group (63% vs 88%). The actuarial survival curves with freedom from combined events at 2 years in the calcified group became significantly poorer as the severity of calcification increased. These findings are in agreement with several follow-up studies of surgical commissurotomy, which demonstrate that patients with calcified mitral valves had a poorer survival compared with those patients with uncalcified valves.[40,43,44]

Follow-Up of Patients with Previous Surgical Commissurotomy

PMV also has been shown to be a safe procedure in patients with previous surgical mitral commissurotomy.[14,24,29,41–46] Although a good immediate outcome is frequently achieved in these patients, follow-up results are not as favorable as those obtained in patients without previous surgical commissurotomy. Although there is no difference in mortality between patients with or without a history of previous surgical commissurotomy at 4-year follow-up, the number of patients who required mitral valve replacement (26% vs 8%) and/or were in NYHA class III or IV (35% vs 13%) was significantly higher among those patients with previous commissurotomy. When the patients are carefully selected according to the echocardiographic score ($\leq$8), however, the immediate outcome and the 4-year follow-up results are excellent and similar to thoseseen in patients without previous surgical commissurotomy.

Follow-Up of Patients with Atrial Fibrillation

The authors have reported that the presence of atrial fibrillation is associated with inferior immediate and long-term outcome after PMV as reflected in a smaller post-PMV MVA and a lower event-free survival (freedom from death, redo-PMV, and mitral valve surgery) at a median follow-up time of 61 months (32% vs 61%; $P<.0001$).[47] Analysis of preprocedural and procedural characteristics revealed that this association is most likely explained by the presence of multiple factors in the atrial fibrillation group that adversely affect the immediate and long-term outcome of PMV. Patients in atrial fibrillation are older and presented more frequently with NYHA class IV, echocardiographic score greater than 8, calcified valves under fluoroscopy, and a history of previous surgical commissurotomy. In the group of patients in atrial fibrillation, the authors identified severe post-PMV MR (>3+) ($P = .0001$), echocardiographic score greater than 8 ($P = .004$), and pre-PMV NYHA class IV ($P = .046$) as independent predictors of combined events at follow-up. The presence of atrial fibrillation per se should not be the only determinant in the decision process regarding treatment options in patients with rheumatic mitral stenosis. The presence of an echocardiographic score less than or equal to 8 primarily identifies a subgroup of patients in atrial fibrillation in whom percutaneous balloon valvotomy is likely to be successful and provide good long-term results. Therefore, in this group of patients, PMV should be the procedure of choice.

Follow-Up of Patients with Pulmonary Artery Hypertension

The degree of pulmonary artery hypertension before PMV is inversely related to the immediate and long-term outcome of PMV.[17,48] Chen and colleagues[49] divided 564 patients undergoing PMV at Massachusetts General Hospital into 3 groups on the basis of the pulmonary vascular resistance (PVR) obtained at cardiac catheterization immediately before PMV: group I with less than or equal to 250 dyne $\cdot$ s $\cdot$ cm^{-5} (normal/mildly elevated resistance) comprised 332 patients (59%); group II with a PVR between 251 and 400 250 dyne $\cdot$ s $\cdot$ cm^{-5} (moderately elevated resistance) comprised 110 patients (19.5%); and group III with a PVR greater than or equal to 400 dyne $\cdot$ s $\cdot$ cm^{-5} comprised 122 patients (21.5%).

Patients in groups I and II were younger and had less severe heart failure symptoms measured by NYHA class and a lower incidence of echocardiographic scores greater than 8, atrial fibrillation, and calcium noted on fluoroscopy than patients in group III. Before and after PMV, patients with higher PVR had a smaller MVA, lower cardiac output, and higher mean pulmonary artery pressure. For groups I, II, and III patients, the immediate success rates for PMV were 68%, 56%, and 45%, respectively. Therefore, patients in the group with severely elevated pulmonary artery resistance before the procedure had lower immediate success rates of PMV. At long-term follow-up, patients with severely elevated pulmonary vascular resistance had a significant lower survival and event-free survival (survival with freedom from mitral valve surgery or NYHA class III or IV heart failure).

Follow-Up of Patients with Tricuspid Regurgitation

The degree of tricuspid regurgitation before PMV is inversely related to the immediate and long-term outcome of PMV. Sagie and colleagues[50] divided patients undergoing PMV at Massachusetts General Hospital into 3 groups on the basis of the degree of tricuspid regurgitation determined by 2-D and color-flow Doppler echocardiography before PMV. Patients with severe tricuspid regurgitation before PMV were older and had more severe heart failure symptoms measured by NYHA class and a higher incidence of echocardiographic scores greater than 8, atrial fibrillation, and calcified mitral valves on fluoroscopy than patients with mild or moderate tricuspid regurgitation. Patients with severe tricuspid regurgitation had a smaller MVAs before and after PMV than the patients with mild or moderate tricuspid regurgitation. At long-term follow-up, patients with severe tricuspid regurgitation had a significant lower survival and event-free survival (survival with freedom from mitral valve surgery or NYHA class III or IV heart failure). The degree of tricuspid regurgitation can be diminished when the transmitral pressure gradient is sufficiently relieved with PMV.[48–50]

Follow-Up of the Best Patients for PMV

In patients identified as optimal candidates for PMV, this technique results in excellent immediate and long-term outcome. Optimal candidates for PMV are those patients meeting the following characteristics: (1) age 45 years old or younger; (2) normal sinus rhythm; (3) echocardiographic score less than or equal to 8; (4) no history of previous surgical commissurotomy; and (5) pre-PMV MR less than or equal to 1+ Sellers grade. From 879 consecutive patients undergoing PMV, the authors identified 136 patients with optimal preprocedure characteristics. In these patients, PMV results in an 81% success rate and a 3.4% incidence of major in-hospital combined events (death and/or MVR). In these patients, PMV results in a 95% survival and 61% event-free survival at 12 years' follow-up.[17,29]

The Double-Balloon Versus the Inoue Techniques of PMV

Today the Inoue approach of PMV is the technique more widely used. There was controversy as to whether the double-balloon or the Inoue technique provided superior immediate and long-term results. The authors compared the immediate procedural and the long-term clinical outcomes after PMV using the double-balloon technique (n = 659) and Inoue technique (n = 233).[52] There were no statistically significant differences in baseline clinical and morphologic characteristics between the double-balloon technique and Inoue technique patients. Although the post-PMV MVA was larger with the double-balloon technique (1.94 ± 0.72 vs 1.81 ± 0.58; $P = .01$), success rate (71.3% vs 69.1%; $P =$ not significant), incidence of greater than 3+ MR (9% vs 9%), in-hospital complications, and long-term and event-free survival were similar with both techniques. In conclusion, both the Inoue and the double-balloon techniques are equally effective techniques of PMV. The procedure of choice should be performed based on the interventionist experience in the technique.

Echocardiographic and Hemodynamic Follow-Up

Follow-up studies have shown that the incidence of hemodynamic and echocardiographic restenosis is low after PMV.[6,17,29,52] A study of a group of patients undergoing simultaneous clinical evaluation, 2-D Doppler echocardiography, and transseptal catheterization 2 years after PMV reported 90% of patients in NYHA classes I and II and 10% of patients in NYHA class III or higher.[52] In this study, hemodynamic determination of MVA using the Gorlin equation showed a significant decrease in MVA from 2.0 cm^2 immediately after PMV to 1.6 cm^2 at follow-up. There was no significant difference, however, between the echocardiographic MVAs immediately after PMV and at follow-up (1.8 cm^2 and 1.6 cm^2, respectively; $P =$ not significant). Although there was a significant difference in the MVA after PMV determined by the Gorlin equation and by 2-D echocardiography (2.0

cm^2 vs 1.8 cm^2), there was no significant difference between the MVA determined by the Gorlin equation and the echocardiographic calculated MVA (1.6 cm^2 for both) at follow-up. The discrepancy between the 2-D echocardiographic and Gorlin equation determined post-PMV MVAs is due to the contribution of left-to-right shunting (undetected by oximetry) across the created interatrial communication, which results in both an erroneously high cardiac output and an overestimation of the MVA by the Gorlin equation.[53] Desideri and colleagues[40] showed no significant differences in MVA (measured by Doppler echocardiography) at 19 ± 6 (range 9–33) months follow-up between the post-PMV and follow-up MVAs. MVAs were 2.2 ± 0.5 cm^2 and 1.9 ± 0.5 cm^2, respectively. Echocardiographic restenosis (MVA ≤1.5 cm^2 with >50% reduction of the gain) was estimated in 39% at 7 years' follow-up with the Inoue technique.[46] A mitral area loss greater than or equal to 0.3 cm^2 was seen in 12%, 22%, and 27% of patients at 3, 5, and 7 years, respectively. Predictors of restenosis included a post-MVA less than 1.8 cm^2 and an echocardiographic score greater than 8.

PMV Versus Surgical Mitral Commissurotomy

Results of surgical closed mitral commissurotomy have demonstrated favorable long-term hemodynamic and symptomatic improvement from this technique. A restenosis rate of 4.2 to 11.4 per 1000 patients per year was reported by John and colleagues[54] in 3724 patients who underwent surgical closed mitral commissurotomy. Survival after PMV is similar to that reported after surgical mitral commissurotomy. Although freedom from mitral valve replacement and freedom from all events after PMV are lower than reported after surgical commissurotomy, freedom from both mitral valve replacement and all events in patients with echocardiographic scores less than or equal to 8 are similar to that reported after surgical mitral commissurotomy.[21–24]

Restenosis after both closed and open surgical mitral commissurotomy has being well documented.[54–56] Although surgical closed mitral commissurotomy is uncommonly performed in the United States, it is still used frequently in other countries. Long-term follow-up of 267 patients who underwent surgical transventricular mitral commissurotomy at the Mayo Clinic showed 79%, 67%, and 55% survival rates at 10, 15, and 20 years, respectively. Survival rates with freedom from mitral valve replacement were 57%, 36%, and 24%, respectively.[57] In this study age, atrial fibrillation and male gender were independent

predictors of death, whereas mitral valve calcification, cardiomegaly, and MR were independent predictors of repeat mitral valve surgery.

Because of similar patient selection and mechanism of mitral valve dilatation, similar long-term results should be expected after PMV. Prospective randomized trials comparing PMV and surgical closed or open mitral commissurotomy have shown no differences in immediate and 3-year follow-up results between both groups of patients.[19–23] Furthermore, restenosis at 3-year follow-up occurred in 10% and 13% of the patients treated with mitral balloon valvuloplasty and surgical commissurotomy, respectively.[19–23]

Interpretation of long-term clinical follow-up of patients undergoing PMV as well as their comparison with surgical commissurotomy series are confounded by heterogeneity in patient populations. Most surgical series have involved a younger population with optimal mitral valve morphology and pliable with no calcification and no evidence of subvalvular disease. Comparisons were also made at the beginning of PMV. Therefore, surgeons were more experienced than interventional cardiologists. Differences in age and valve morphology may also account for the lower survival and event-free survival of PMV series from the United States and Europe.[29,44]

Several studies have compared the immediate and early follow-up results of PMV versus closed surgical commissurotomy in optimal patients for these techniques. The results of these studies have been controversial showing either superior outcome from PMV or no significant differences between both techniques.[19–23] Patel and colleagues[18] randomized 45 patients with mitral stenosis and optimal mitral valve morphology to closed surgical commissurotomy and to PMV. They demonstrated a larger increase in MVA with PMV (2.1 ± 0.7 vs 1.3 ± 0.3 cm^2). Shrivastava and colleagues[19] compared the results of single-balloon PMV, double-balloon PMV, and closed surgical commissurotomy in 3 groups of 20 patients each. The MVA postintervention was larger for the double-balloon technique of PMV. Postintervention valve areas were 1.9 ± 0.8, 1.5 ± 0.4, and 1.5 ± 0.5 for the double-balloon, single-balloon, and closed surgical commissurotomy techniques, respectively. Alternatively, Arora and colleagues[20] randomized 200 patients with a mean age of 19 ± 7 years and mitral stenosis with optimal mitral valve morphology to PMV and to closed mitral commissurotomy. Both procedures resulted in similar postintervention MVAs (2.39 ± 0.9 vs 2.2 ± 0.9 cm^2 for the PMV and the mitral commissurotomy groups, respectively) and no significant differences in event-free survival at a mean follow-up period of 22 ± 6 months. Restenosis documented by echocardiography was low in both groups, 5% in the PMV group, and 4% in the closed commissurotomy group. Turi and colleagues[21] randomized 40 patients with severe mitral stenosis to PMV and to closed surgical commissurotomy. The postintervention MVA at 1 week (1.6 ± 0.6 vs 1.6 ± 0.7 cm²) and 8 months (1.6 ± 0.6 vs 1.8 ± 0.6 cm²) after the procedures were similar in both groups. Reyes and colleagues[22] randomized 60 patients with severe mitral stenosis and favorable valvular anatomy to PMV and to surgical commissurotomy. They reported no significant differences in immediate outcome, complications, and 3.5 years' follow-up between both groups of patients. Improvement was maintained in both groups, but MVAs at follow-up were larger in the PMV group (2.4 ± 0.6 vs 1.8 ± 0.4 cm²). Ben Farhat and colleagues[23] reported the results of a randomized trial designed to compare the immediate and long-term results of double-balloon PMV with those of open and closed surgical mitral commissurotomy in a cohort of patients with severe rheumatic mitral stenosis. These patients were, from clinical and morphologic points of view, optimal candidates for both PMV and surgical commissurotomy (closed or open) procedures. They had a mean age of less than 30 years, absence of mitral valve calcification on fluoroscopy and 2-D echocardiography, and an echocardiographic score less than or equal to 8 in all patients. Their results demonstrate that the immediate and long-term results of PMV are comparable to those of open mitral commissurotomy and superior to those of closed commissurotomy. The hemodynamic improvement, in-hospital complications, and long-term restenosis rate and need for reintervention were superior for the patients treated with either PMV or open commissurotomy than for those treated with closed commissurotomy. The postintervention MVAs achieved with PMV were similar to the one obtained after open surgical commissurotomy (2.5 ± 0.5 vs 2.2 ± 0.4 cm²) but larger than those obtained after closed commissurotomy. These initial changes resulted in an excellent long-term follow-up in the group of patients treated with PMV, which was comparable with the open commissurotomy group and superior to the closed commissurotomy group. The inferior results of closed mitral commissurotomy presented by Ben Farhat and colleagues are in disagreement with previous studies showing no significant differences in immediate and follow-up results between PMV and closed surgical mitral commissurotomy.[18–21] The increase in MVA after closed commissurotomy, however, is not uniform and often unsatisfactory. Because open commissurotomy is associated with a thoracotomy, need for cardiopulmonary bypass, higher cost, longer length of hospital stay, and a longer period of convalescence, PMV should be the procedure of choice for the treatment of patients with rheumatic mitral stenosis who are, from clinical and morphologic points of view, optimal candidates for PMV.[17,24,29]

PMV in Pregnant Women

Surgical mitral commissurotomy has been performed in pregnant women with severe mitral stenosis. Because the risk of anesthesia and surgery for the mother and the fetus are increased, this operation is reserved for those patients with incapacitating symptoms refractory to medical therapy.[58–60] Under these conditions, PMV can be performed safely after the twentieth week of pregnancy with minimal radiation to the fetus.[58–60] Because of the definite risk in women with severe mitral stenosis of developing symptoms during pregnancy, PMV should be considered when a patient is considering becoming pregnant.

Difference in Outcome among Women and Men after Percutaneous Mitral Valvuloplasty

The authors evaluated measures of procedural success and clinical outcome in 1015 consecutive patients (839 women and 176 men) who underwent PMV. Despite a lower baseline echocardiographic score (7.47 ± 2.15 vs 8.02 ± 2.18; P = .002), women were less likely to achieve PMV success (69% vs 83%; adjusted OR 0.44; 95% CI, 0.27–0.74; P = .002) and had a smaller postprocedural MV area (1.86 ± 0.7 vs 2.07 ± 0.7 cm²; P<.001). Overall procedural and in-hospital complication rates did not differ significantly between women and men. Women, however, were significantly more likely to develop severe MR immediately post-PMV (adjusted OR 2.41; 95% CI, 1.0–5.83; P = .05) and to undergo MV surgery (adjusted hazard ratio 1.54; 95% CI, 1.03–2.3; P = .037) after a median follow-up of 3.1 years. Thus, compared with men, women with rheumatic mitral stenosis who undergo PMV are less likely to have a successful outcome and more likely to require MV surgery on long-term follow-up despite more favorable baseline mitral valve anatomy.[61]

SUMMARY

PMV should be the procedure of choice for the treatment of patients with rheumatic mitral stenosis who are, from clinical and morphologic points of view, optimal candidates for PMV.[17] Patients with echocardiographic scores less than or equal to 8 have the best results, particularly if they are young, are in sinus rhythm, have no pulmonary hypertension, and have no evidence of calcification of the mitral valve under fluoroscopy. The immediate and long-term results of PMV in this group of patients are similar to those reported after surgical mitral commissurotomy.[17] Patients with echocardiographic scores greater than 8 have only a 50% chance to obtain a successful hemodynamic result with PMV, and long-term follow-up results are less good than those from patients with echocardiographic scores less than or equal to 8. In patients with echocardiographic scores greater than or equal to 12, it is unlikely that PMV could produce good immediate or long-term results. They preferably should undergo open heart surgery. PMV could be performed in these patients if they are non-high risk surgical candidates. Finally, much remains to be done in refining indications for patients with few or no symptoms and those with unfavorable anatomy. Surgical therapy for mitral stenosis should be reserved, however, for patients who have greater than or equal to 2 Sellers grades of MR by angiography, which can be better treated by mitral valve repair, and for those patients with severe mitral valve thickening and calcification or with significant subvalvular scarring to warrant valve replacement.[17]

REFERENCES

1. Inoue K, Owaki T, Nakamura T, et al. Clinical application of transvenous mitral commissurotomy by a new balloon catheter. J Thorac Cardiovasc Surg 1984;87: 394–402.
2. Lock JE, Kalilullah M, Shrivastava S, et al. Percutaneous catheter commissurotomy in rheumatic mitral stenosis. N Engl J Med 1985;313:1515–8.
3. Al Zaibag M, Ribeiro PA, Al Kassab SA, et al. Percutaneous double balloon mitral valvotomy for rheumatic mitral stenosis. Lancet 1986;1:757–61.
4. Palacios I, Block PC, Brandi S, et al. Percutaneous balloon valvotomy for patients with severe mitral stenosis. Circulation 1987;75:778–84.
5. Mc Kay CR, Kawanishi DT, Rahimtoola SH. Catheter balloon valvuloplasty of the mitral valve in adults using a double balloon technique. Early hemodynamic results. JAMA 1987;257:1753–61.
6. Cohen DJ, Kuntz RE, Gordon SP, et al. Predictors of long-term outcome after percutaneous mitral valvuloplasty. N Engl J Med 1991;327:1329–35.
7. Arora R, Kalra GS, Murty GS, et al. Percutaneous transatrial mitral commissurotomy: immediate and intermediate results. J Am Coll Cardiol 1994;23: 1327–32.
8. Chen CR, Cheng TO. Percutaneous balloon mitral valvuloplasty by the Inoue technique: a multicenter

study of 4832 patients in China. Am Heart J 1995; 129:1197–203.
9. Dean LS, Mickel M, Bonan R, et al. Four-year follow-up of patients undergoing percutaneous balloon mitral commissurotomy. A report from the National Heart, Lung, and Blood Institute Balloon Valvuloplasty Registry. J Am Coll Cardiol 1996; 28:1452–7.
10. Orrange SE, Kawanishi DT, Lopez BM, et al. Actuarial outcome after catheter balloon commissurotomy in patients with mitral stenosis. Circulation 1997;97:245–50.
11. Chen CR, Cheng TO, Chen JY, et al. Long-term results of percutaneous balloon mitral valvuloplasty for mitral stenosis: a follow-up study to 11 years in 202 patients. Cathet Cardiovasc Diagn 1998;43: 132–9.
12. Stefanadis CI, Stratos CG, Lambrou SG, et al. Retrograde nontransseptal balloon mitral valvuloplasty: immediate results and intermediate long-term outcome in 441 cases–a multicenter experience. J Am Coll Cardiol 1998;32:1009–16.
13. Cribier A, Eltchaninoff H, Koning R, et al. Percutaneous mechanical mitral commissurotomy with a newly designed metallic valvulotome: immediate results of the initial experience in 153 patients. Circulation 1999;99:793–9.
14. Hernandez R, Banuelos C, Alfonso F, et al. Long-term clinical and echocardiographic follow-up after percutaneous mitral valvuloplasty with the Inoue balloon. Circulation 1999;99:1580–6.
15. Iung B, Garbarz E, Michaud P, et al. Late results of percutaneous mitral commissurotomy in a series of 1024 patients: analysis of late clinical deterioration: frequency, anatomic findings and predictive factors. Circulation 1999;99:3272–8.
16. Cribier A, Eltchaninoff H, Carlot R, et al. Percutaneous mechanical mitral commissurotomy with the metallic valvulotome: detailed technical aspects and overview of the results of the multicenter registry in 882 patients. J Interv Cardiol 2000;13:255–62.
17. Palacios IF, Sanchez PL, Harrell LC, et al. Which patients benefit from percutaneous mitral balloon valvuloplasty? Prevalvuloplasty and postvalvuloplasty variables that predict long-term outcome. Circulation 2002;105:1465–71.
18. Patel JJ, Shama D, Mitha AS, et al. Balloon valvuloplasty versus closed commissurotomy for pliable mitral stenosis: a prospective hemodynamic study. J Am Coll Cardiol 1991;18:1318–22.
19. Shrivastava S, Mathur A, Dev V, et al. A comparison of immediate hemodynamic response of closed mitral commissurotomy, single-balloon, and double-balloon mitral valvuloplasty in rheumatic mitral stenosis. J Thorac Cardiovasc Surg 1992;104:1264–7.
20. Arora R, Nair M, Kalra GS, et al. Immediate and long-term results of balloon and surgical closed

mitral valvotomy: a randomized comparative study. Am Heart J 1993;125:1091–4.

21. Turi ZG, Reyes VP, Raju BS, et al. Percutaneous balloon versus surgical closed commissurotomy for mitral stenosis: a prospective, randomized trial. Circulation 1991;83:1179–85.

22. Reyes VP, Raju BS, Wynne J, et al. Percutaneous balloon valvuloplasty compared with open surgical commissurotomy for mitral stenosis. N Engl J Med 1994;331:961–7.

23. Ben Farhat M, Ayari M, Maatouk F, et al. Percutaneous balloon versus surgical closed and open mitral commissurotomy: seven-year follow-up results of a randomized trial. Circulation 1998; 97:245–50.

24. Babic UU, Pejcic P, Djurisic Z, et al. Percutaneous transarterial balloon valvuloplasty for mitral valve stenosis. Am J Cardiol 1986;57:1101–4.

25. Stefanadis C, Stratos C, Pitsavos C, et al. Retrograde nontransseptal balloon mitral valvuloplasty. Immediate results and long term follow-up. Circulation 1992;85:1760–7.

26. Cruz-Gonzalez I, Sanchez-Ledesma M, Sanchez PL, et al. Predicting success and long-term outcomes of percutaneous mitral valvuloplasty: a multifactorial score. Am J Med 2009;122:581–90.

27. Mc Kay RG, Lock JE, Safian RD, et al. Balloon dilatation of mitral stenosis in adults patients: postmortem and percutaneous mitral valvuloplasty studies. J Am Coll Cardiol 1987;9:723–31.

28. Herrmann HC, Lima JA, Feldman T, et al. Mechanisms and outcome of severe mitral regurgitation after Inoue balloon valvuloplasty. J Am Coll Cardiol 1993;27:783–9.

29. Padial LR, Freitas N, Sagie A, et al. Echocardiography can predict which patients will develop severe mitral regurgitation after precutaneous mitral valvulotomy. J Am Coll Cardiol 1996;27:1225–31.

30. Palacios IF. Farewell to surgical mitral commissurotomy for many patients. Circulation 1998;97:223–6.

31. Abascal VM, O'Shea JP, Wilkins GT, et al. Prediction of successful outcome in 130 patients undergoing percutaneous balloon mitral valvotomy. Circulation 1990;82:448–56.

32. Herrmann HC, Wilkins GT, Abascal VM, et al. Percutaneous balloon mitral valvotomy for patients with mitral stenosis: analysis of factors influencing early results. J Thorac Cardiovasc Surg 1988;96:33–8.

33. Wilkins GT, Weyman AE, Abascal VM, et al. Percutaneous balloon dilatation of the mitral valve: an analysis of echocardiographic variables related to outcome and the mechanism of dilatation. Br Heart J 1988;60:229–308.

34. Abascal VM, Wilkins GT, Choong CY, et al. Mitral regurgitation after percutaneous mitral valvuloplasty in adults: evaluation by pulsed Doppler echocardiography. J Am Coll Cardiol 1988;2:257–63.

35. Roth RB, Block PC, Palacios IF. Predictors of increased mitral regurgitation after percutaneous mitral balloon valvotomy. Cathet Cardiovasc Diagn 1990;20:17–21.

36. Tuzcu EM, Block PC, Griffin BP, et al. Immediate and long term outcome of percutaneous mitral valvotomy in patients 65 years and older. Circulation 1992;85:963–71.

37. Sánchez PL, Rodríguez-Alemparte M, Inglessis I, et al. The impact of age in the immediate and long-term outcomes of percutaneous mitral balloon valvuloplasty. J Invasive Cardiol 2005;18(4):217–25.

38. Sellers RD, Levy MJ, Amplatz K, et al. Left retrograde cardioangiography in acquired cardiac disease. Am J Cardiol 1964;14:437–47.

39. Casale P, Block PC, O'Shea JP, et al. Atrial septal defect after percutaneous mitral balloon valvuloplasty: immediate results and follow-up. J Am Coll Cardiol 1990;15:1300–4.

40. Desideri A, Vanderperren O, Serra A, et al. Long term (9 to 33 months) echocardiographic follow-up after successful percutaneous mitral commissurotomy. Am J Cardiol 1992;69:1602–6.

41. Tuzcu EM, Block PC, Griffin B, et al. Percutaneous mitral balloon valvotomy in patients with calcific mitral stenosis: immediate and long term outcome. J Am Coll Cardiol 1994;23:1604–9.

42. Rediker DE, Block PC, Abascal VM, et al. Mitral balloon valvuloplasty for mitral restenosis after surgical commissurotomy. J Am Coll Cardiol 1988; 2:252–6.

43. Medina A, Suarez De Lezo J, Hernandez E, et al. Balloon valvuloplasty for mitral restenosis after previous surgery. A comparative study. Am Heart J 1990;120:568–71.

44. Davidson CJ, Bashore TM, Mickel M, et al. Balloon mitral commissurotomy after previous surgical commissurotomy. The National Heart, Lung, and Blood Institute balloon valvuloplasty registry participants. Circulation 1992;86:91–9.

45. Vahanian A, Palacios IF. Percutaneous approaches to valvular disease. Circulation 2004;109:1572–9.

46. Jang IK, Block PC, Newell JB, et al. Percutaneous mitral balloon valvotomy for recurrent mitral stenosis after surgical commissurotomy. Am J Cardiol 1995; 75:601–5.

47. Lau KW, Ding ZP, Gao W, et al. Percutaneous balloon mitral valvuloplasty in patients with mitral restenosis after previous surgical commissurotomy. A matched comparative study. Eur Heart J 1996; 17:1367–72.

48. Leon MN, Harrell LC, Simosa HF, et al. Mitral balloon valvotomy for patients with mitral stenosis in atrial fibrillation: immediate and long-term results. J Am Coll Cardiol 1999;34:1145–52.

49. Chen MH, Semigran M, Schwammenthal E, et al. Impact of pulmonary resistance on short and long

term outcome after percutaneous mitral valvuloplasty. Circulation 1993;(Suppl 1):1825.

50. Sagie A, Schwammenthal E, Newell JB, et al. Significant tricuspid regurgitation is a marker for adverse outcome in patients undergoing mitral balloon valvotomy. J Am Coll Cardiol 1994;24:696–702.

51. Song JM, Kang DH, Song JK, et al. Outcome of significant functional tricuspid regurgitation after percutaneous mitral valvuloplasty. Am Heart J 2003;145:371–6.

52. Sanchez PL, Harrell LC, Salas RE, et al. Learning curve of the Inoue technique of percutaneous mitral balloon valvuloplasty. Am J Cardiol 2001;88:662–7.

53. Block PC, Palacios IF, Block EH, et al. Late (two year) follow-up after percutaneous mitral balloon valvotomy. Am J Cardiol 1992;69:537–41.

54. Petrossian GA, Tuzcu EM, Ziskind AA, et al. Atrial septal occlusion improves the accuracy of mitral valve area determination following percutaneous mitral balloon valvotomy. Cathet Cardiovasc Diagn 1991;22:21–4.

55. John S, Bashi VV, Jairaj PS, et al. Closed mitral valvotomy: early results and long term follow up of 3724 patients. Circulation 1983;68:891–6.

56. Ellis LR, Harken DE, Black H. A clinical study of 1,000 consecutive cases of mitral stenosis two to nine years after mitral valvuloplasty. Circulation 1959;19:803–20.

57. Rihal CS, Schaff HV, Frye RL, et al. Long-term follow-up of patients undergoing closed transventricular mitral commissurotomy: a useful surrogate for percutaneous balloon mitral valvuloplasty. J Am Coll Cardiol 1992;20:781–6.

58. Palacios IF, Block PC, Wilkins GT, et al. Percutaneous mitral balloon valvotomy during pregnancy in patients with severe mitral stenosis. Cathet Cardiovasc Diagn 1988;15:109–11.

59. Mangione JA, Zuliani MF, Del Castillo JM, et al. Percutaneous double balloon mitral valvuloplasty in pregnant women. Am J Cardiol 1989;64:99–102.

60. Esteves C, Munoz JS, Sergio Braga S, et al. Immediate and long-term follow-up of percutaneous balloon mitral valvuloplasty in pregnant patients with rheumatic mitral stenosis. Am J Cardiol 2006;98:812–6.

61. Cruz-Gonzalez I, Jneid H, Sanchez-Ledesma M, et al. Difference in outcome among women and men after percutaneous mitral valvuloplasty. Cathet Cardiovasc Diagn 2011;77:115–20.

62. Post JR, Feldman T, Isner J, Herrmann HC. Inoue balloon mitral valvotomy in patients with severe valvular and subvalvular deformity. J AM Coll Cardiol 1995;25:1129–36.

Percutaneous Treatment of Mitral Regurgitation: The MitraClip Experience

Alice Perlowski, MD[a], Ted Feldman, MD, FESC, FSCAI[b],*

KEYWORDS

- Mitral regurgitation • Mitral valve repair
- Percutaneous valve therapy • MitraClip • EVEREST Trial

Mitral regurgitation (MR) is the most common type of heart valve disease, affecting approximately 2% of the US population. Available medical therapy is limited in its scope and efficacy. Surgical intervention is the current standard of care of patients who are symptomatic, particularly if the etiology of MR is degenerative. Mitral valve repair, rather than replacement, is associated with excellent durability, lower rates of thromboembolism and infection, and improved survival, and is the surgical approach of choice in suitable candidates.[1]

Patients with prior coronary artery bypass graft surgery, various comorbidities, and older age represent a sizable proportion of patients with severe symptomatic MR. The elevated risk of surgical mortality in this group often precludes operative referral or treatment. A clear need for less-invasive approaches for the treatment of MR for higher-risk patients led to the development of several percutaneous, catheter-based technologies. These include indirect and direct annuloplasty devices, as well as an implantable clip. Currently, all percutaneous therapies for MR are investigational in the United States.

The MitraClip system (Abbott Vascular, Santa Clara, CA, USA) involves an implantable clip applied to the mitral leaflets, replicating a surgical procedure in which the free edges of the mitral leaflets are sutured together to create a double-orifice mitral opening (**Figs. 1** and **2**). The MitraClip is the only percutaneous therapy for MR that has been evaluated in a randomized trial compared with surgical intervention, and it is the most widely applied percutaneous therapy for MR worldwide.

MITRACLIP SYSTEM: HISTORICAL PERSPECTIVE

In 1992, Otavio Alfieri and colleagues[2] described a technique where the mitral leaflet mal-coaptation was corrected by placing a surgical suture to approximate the mid portion of the anterior and posterior leaflets. This "edge-to-edge" technique is usually applied to the A2-P2 central segment of the leaflets, creating a double orifice and reducing MR. Results up to 12 years in patients treated with surgical edge-to-edge repair have been reported.[3]

Alfieri and colleagues' approach for mitral valve repair was the inspiration for the MitraClip, a novel catheter-based system designed to mimic the operative procedure. In 1998, interventional cardiologist Fred St Goar and colleagues[4] developed a percutaneous, catheter-delivered implantable clip, applied to the mitral valve via femoral vein and trans-septal access. The clip and steerable catheter delivery system were initially tested in the porcine model, where postmortem analysis confirmed creation of a double orifice and correct

Disclosures: Dr Feldman is a consult for and receives research grants from Abbott, Boston Scientific, and Edwards. Dr Perlowski has nothing to disclose.
a NorthShore University HealthSystem, Evanston, IL, USA
b Cardiac Catheterization Laboratory, NorthShore University HealthSystem, Evanston Hospital, 2650 Ridge Avenue, Burch Building, Evanston, IL 60201, USA
* Corresponding author. Cardiology Division, Evanston Hospital, Walgreen Building 3rd Floor, 2650 Ridge Avenue, Evanston, IL 60201.
E-mail address: tfeldman@northshore.org

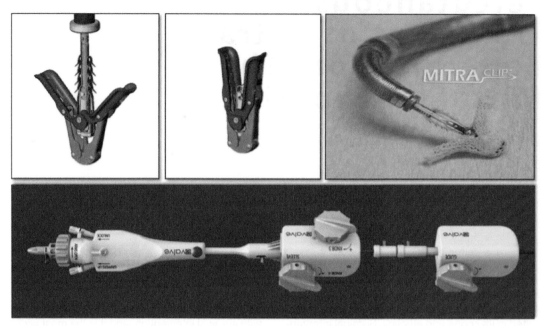

Fig. 1. The Evalve MitraClip. The upper panel shows the clip itself. The clip arms are open when the device is passed across the mitral leaflets from the left atrium into the left ventricle. The gripper is the barbed piece seen in the upper left, parallel to the shaft of the delivery system. When the leaflets are grasped, the gripper helps to fix the leaflets within the clip arms. The clip is covered with polyester fabric. The lower part of the figure shows the steering knobs on the right-hand side of the device for maneuvering the clip within the left atrial cavity. At the far left of the picture is the knob that is used to open and close the clip, and the release mechanism. (*From* Feldman T, Cilingiroglu M. Percutaneous leaflet repair and annuloplasty for mitral regurgitation. J Am Coll Cardiol 2011;57:529–37; with permission.)

deployment perpendicular to the line of coaptation in most animal subjects.

Animal model studies investigating the healing response over time demonstrated that the clip is stable and durable.[5,6] Scanning electron microscopy at 24 weeks showed no evidence of thromboembolism or mitral stenosis. There was clip encapsulation with complete endothelialization,

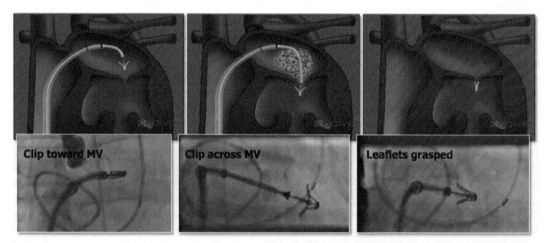

Fig. 2. The basic steps of the Evalve MitraClip clip procedure. The left-hand panel shows the clip being steered through the left atrium toward the center of the mitral orifice. The middle panel illustrates the device across the mitral valve with the clip arms open, before the clip has been pulled back to grasp the mitral leaflets. On the right upper panel, in the illustration, the clip has been released. In the fluoroscopic figure (*right lower*) the leaflets have been grasped and clipped closed partially, before full closure and release of the clip. (*From* Feldman T, Cilingiroglu M. Percutaneous leaflet repair and annuloplasty for mitral regurgitation. J Am Coll Cardiol 2011;57:529–37; with permission.)

followed by formation of a tissue bridge.[5] The tissue bridge created when the clipped segment heals, likely anchors the mitral leaflets together and tethers the annulus in the septal-lateral dimension, possibly preventing additional annular dilatation. A similar healing response has been seen in patients.[7]

The first MitraClip implant in a human subject was performed in Caracas, Venezuela, in June 2003.[8] The patient was a 49-year-old woman who suffered from bileaflet flail and severe, symptomatic MR. The clip was successfully deployed, reducing her MR to less than 2+. The patient's symptoms resolved completely, and follow-up echocardiograms demonstrated stable MR grade, and normalization of left ventricular dimensions and ejection fraction at 2-year follow-up. The first case in the United States was performed several days later at Evanston Hospital, Evanston, Illinois, as part of the initial EVEREST (Endovascular Valve Edge-to-Edge Repair Study) Phase I registry.

CLINICAL OUTCOMES
The EVEREST Trials

Outcomes of therapy with the MitraClip device have been evaluated in the United States in the EVEREST registry, EVEREST II Randomized Trial, and EVEREST II High-Risk Registry. Patients continue to be enrolled in REALISM, the continued access registry of EVEREST II. The total number of patients enrolled in these trials exceeds 1000, rendering the MitraClip the most well investigated percutaneous device for treatment of MR.

EVEREST I

The initial EVEREST cohort was a prospective, multicenter phase I trial designed to evaluate the safety and feasibility of the MitraClip procedure.[9] Anatomically suitable symptomatic patients with moderate to severe (3+) or severe (4+) MR, meeting the American Heart Association/American College of Cardiology guideline recommendations[10] for surgical mitral valve repair, were enrolled (**Box 1**). Prospective qualification of patients occurred based on strict predefined anatomic criteria. Optimal anatomy included a discrete MR jet, originating within the central two-thirds of the line of leaflet coaptation. The degree of mitral valve calcification in the grasping area, flail width, flail gap, coaptation length, coaptation depth, and degree of concomitant mitral stenosis were also carefully assessed (**Fig. 3**). All echocardiograms were evaluated in an echo-core laboratory before patient enrollment.

The initial cohort enrolled a total of 107 patients. Degenerative or combined degenerative and functional MR was present in 79% of patients, with the remainder having pure functional MR. Mean MR grade was 3.3 ± 0.7 at baseline. Successful clip placement occurred in 90% of patients; 2 clips were required in 32%.

Results

Acute procedural success, defined as placement of 1 or more clips resulting in 2+ or lower MR, was 74%. Of the 107 registry patients, 96 (90%) achieved a reduction in MR from the clip or mitral valve surgery performed after a clip attempt. Approximately three-quarters of patients had improvement in clinical symptoms. At 3-year follow-up, 70% of patients remained free of surgical intervention. Eighty-four percent of the surgical procedures performed after clip placement were successful.

The overall major adverse event rate was 9%. Blood transfusions of 2 units or more represented the most of these events. Postprocedure death, prolonged mechanical ventilation, and periprocedural stroke represented less-common adverse events, each affecting fewer than 1%. Partial clip detachment (detachment of a single leaflet from the clip) occurred in 9%, most of which were asymptomatic and detected on 30-day echocardiography. Most partial clip detachments were successfully treated with mitral valve surgery. There were no clip embolizations.

Summary

The EVEREST I registry provided the initial evidence that percutaneous edge-to-edge repair was efficacious and safe. The therapy was effective at reducing MR to 2+ or lower in most patients. The reduction in MR was accompanied by significant clinical improvements, with New York Heart Association (NYHA) Class III/IV symptoms decreasing from 55% at baseline to 8% at 12 months.

The MitraClip procedure was also remarkably safe: there were no intraprocedure and minimal periprocedural complications and low rates of major and minor adverse events. The procedure was well tolerated. Manipulation of a device in the mitral orifice with a beating heart did not result in significant hemodynamic derangements, allowing operators to focus on appropriate delivery of the clip, rather than an unstable patient. Hospitalizations were brief, and extubation was possible within the first 24 hours in most patients.

EVEREST investigators appreciated during this initial experience that there was a significant learning curve associated with MitraClip implantation procedures. Most of the cases included in the registry represented the first 3 implantations

Box 1
Indications for mitral valve operation: valve disease guidelines 2008

CLASS I

1. Mitral valve surgery is recommended for the symptomatic patient with acute severe mitral regurgitation (MR) (level of evidence: B).

2. Mitral valve surgery is beneficial for patients with chronic severe MR and New York Heart Association (NYHA) functional class II, III, or IV symptoms in the absence of severe left ventricular (LV) dysfunction (severe LV dysfunction is defined as ejection fraction <0.30) and/or end-systolic dimension larger than 55 mm (level of evidence: B).

3. Mitral valve surgery is beneficial for asymptomatic patients with chronic severe MR and mild-to-moderate LV dysfunction, ejection fraction 0.30 to 0.60, and/or end-systolic dimension of 40 mm or larger (level of evidence: B).

4. Mitral valve repair is recommended over mitral valve replacement in most patients with severe chronic MR who require surgery, and patients should be referred to surgical centers experienced in mitral valve repair (level of evidence: C).

CLASS IIa

1. Mitral valve repair is reasonable in experienced surgical centers for asymptomatic patients with chronic severe MR with preserved LV function (ejection fraction >0.60 and end-systolic dimension <40 mm) in whom the likelihood of successful repair without residual MR is >90% (level of evidence: B).

2. Mitral valve surgery is reasonable for asymptomatic patients with chronic severe MR, preserved LV function, and new onset of atrial fibrillation (level of evidence: C).

3. Mitral valve surgery is reasonable for asymptomatic patients with chronic severe MR, preserved LV function, and pulmonary hypertension (pulmonary artery systolic pressure >50 mm Hg at rest or >60 mm Hg with exercise) (level of evidence: C).

4. Mitral valve surgery is reasonable for patients with chronic severe MR caused by a primary abnormality of the mitral apparatus and NYHA functional class III–IV symptoms and severe LV dysfunction (ejection fraction <0.30 and/or end-systolic dimension >55 mm) in whom mitral valve repair is highly likely (level of evidence: C).

CLASS IIb

1. Mitral valve repair may be considered for patients with chronic severe secondary MR caused by severe LV dysfunction (ejection fraction <0.30) who have persistent NYHA functional class III–IV symptoms despite optimal therapy for heart failure, including biventricular pacing (level of evidence: C).

CLASS III

1. Mitral valve surgery is not indicated for asymptomatic patients with MR and preserved LV function (ejection fraction >0.60 and end-systolic dimension <40 mm) in whom significant doubt about the feasibility of repair exists (level of evidence: C).

2. Isolated mitral valve surgery is not indicated for patients with mild or moderate MR (level of evidence: C).

Data from Bonow RO, Carabello BA, Chatterjee K, et al. 2008 focused update incorporated into the ACC/AHA 2006 guidelines for the management of patients with valvular heart disease: a report of the American College of Cardiology/American Heart Association Task Force on Practice Guidelines (Writing Committee to Develop Guidelines for the Management of Patients With Valvular Heart Disease. J Am Coll Cardiol 2008;52:e1–142.

performed at respective centers. With increasing experience, operators clearly became more proficient with the device. In EVEREST I, procedure times in the final one-third of the cohort were almost an hour shorter than procedures in the first third of the cohort. Device success rates have continued to improve from 90% in the early experience to 98% in the most recent continued access registry experience.

It became clear from the EVEREST I registry experience that careful evaluation of mitral valve anatomy was critical for optimal patient selection. It is crucial that the operator understand the composition and orientation of the mitral valve leaflets and the location of the mitral regurgitant jet before the procedure to ensure that clip implantation is feasible. For patients with functional MR, key inclusion criteria in the EVEREST I registry

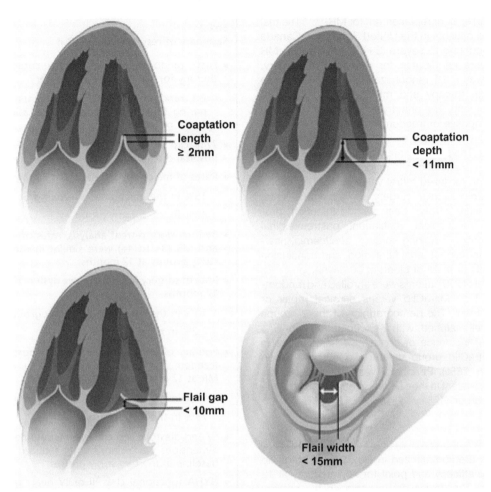

Fig. 3. Echocardiographic evaluation of morphology of mitral leaflets is critical for good patient selection. (*Top*) A coaptation length of at least 2 mm is needed. Thus, some tissue from both leaflets should be in contact, so there is some tissue to grasp with the clip. The coaptation depth should be <11 mm. (*Bottom*) With a flail mitral leaflet, a flail gap of 10 mm and a flail width on short-axis estimation of 15 mm are also important anatomic features. The MR jet must arise from the central two-thirds of the line of coaptation, as seen on short-axis color Doppler examination. Figure illustration by Craig Skaggs. (*From* Feldman T, Cilingiroglu M. Percutaneous leaflet repair and annuloplasty for mitral regurgitation. J Am Coll Cardiol 2011;57:529–37; with permission.)

included a coaptation length of 2 mm or longer and a coaptation depth of 11 mm or more. For patients with leaflet flail, a flail gap less than 10 mm and flail width less than 15 mm was required (see **Fig. 3**). In all patients, the origin of the MR jet was within the central two-thirds of the line of coaptation in the short-axis color Doppler examination. Patients with mitral stenosis (mitral valve orifice area smaller than 4 cm^2) were excluded, as were those with significant calcification within the clipping zone.

This detailed anatomic information is obtained from a quality transthoracic echocardiogram with extensive interrogation of the mitral valve in multiple views, particularly in the parasternal short axis. In EVEREST I, echocardiograms were performed and evaluated in a central, core laboratory. In centers continuing to perform MitraClip therapy, a clear communication must be present between interventionalists, noninvasive cardiologists, and echo technologists to ensure that screening echocardiograms are performed and evaluated with these criteria in mind to ensure that patient selection is optimal.

EVEREST II randomized trial

The EVEREST I registry introduced MitraClip as one of several promising percutaneous therapies for the treatment of MR, but did not address how the catheter-based approach compared with surgical intervention. EVEREST II was a multi-center, randomized controlled trial designed to evaluate the safety and efficacy of percutaneous mitral repair with the MitraClip versus conventional surgical repair or replacement for MR.[11,12] The trial enrolled patients in the United States and Canada with moderate to severe (3+) or severe (4+) MR who were candidates for mitral valve surgery. There was a 2:1 randomization scheme between MitraClip therapy and mitral surgery (repair or replacement). The primary efficacy end point was the composite of freedom from surgery for mitral valve dysfunction, 3 or 4+ MR, and death at 12 months. The primary safety end point was defined as a composite of death, myocardial infarction, re-operation for failed mitral valve surgery, nonelective cardiovascular surgery for adverse events, renal failure, stroke, deep wound infection, prolonged mechanical ventilation, gastrointestinal complication requiring surgery, septicemia, new-onset permanent atrial fibrillation, and transfusion of 2 units or more of blood at 30 days.

A total of 279 patients were enrolled and randomized 2:1 to MitraClip versus surgical repair or replacement. The demographics of the 2 groups were well matched, with 2 exceptions. There was a higher incidence of congestive heart failure in the MitraClip group versus the surgical group (91% vs 78%). Peripheral vascular disease was more prevalent in the surgical group versus the MitraClip group (12% vs 7%).

Results

Results are summarized in **Box 2**. The MitraClip met the efficacy end point for noninferiority at 12 months. The device group achieved the primary efficacy end point (composite freedom from death, surgery for mitral valve dysfunction, or 3 or 4+ MR) in 55% compared with 73% in the surgical group (P = .0007) in an intention-to-treat analysis. The increased rate of surgical referral after MitraClip therapy drove the difference in this composite end point: the need for subsequent surgery was 20% in the MitraClip group at 12 months, compared with 2.2% for repeat mitral valve surgery in the surgical group. Importantly, the frequency of death and MR grade 3 or 4+ was not different in the device versus the surgical group, and 80% of the MitraClip recipients avoided surgery in the first 12 months.

The MitraClip continued to meet its efficacy end point for noninferiority at 2 years (P = .04), with surgery being superior for better reduction in MR grade. The difference in composite end point was again weighted by the increased need for surgery for valve dysfunction after the procedure in the percutaneous group (22% vs 4% in the surgical group). The number of patients receiving MitraClip therapy remaining free of surgical intervention at 2-year follow-up remained close to 80%.

Box 2
Summary of results of EVEREST II

- First randomized trial of percutaneous therapy for MR compared to surgery
  - 2:1 randomization of 279 patients comparing MitraClip to conventional surgical repair or replacement
- 77% clip treated patients with <2+ MR at hospital discharge
- Rates of major adverse events at 30 days
  - 15% in the percutaneous-repair group
  - 48% in the surgery group
- By intention-to-treat analysis, rates of death and MR (3+ to 4+) were similar in the two study groups at 12 months
- Rate of surgery for mitral-valve dysfunction at 12 months
  - 20% in the percutaneous-repair group
  - 2.2% in the surgery group
- Primary efficacy end point (a composite of freedom from death, surgery and 3+ to 4+ MR at 12 months)
  - 55% in the percutaneous-repair group
  - 73% in the surgery group, P = .007
- LV end-diastolic and end-systolic volumes and dimensions were significantly reduced from baseline in the two study groups
- NYHA functional class III or IV heart failure present in
  - 2% of patients in the percutaneous repair group
  - 13% of those in the surgery group, P = .002
- Subgroups that had the best results with percutaneous repair were
  - >70 years
  - LVEF<60%
  - functional MR
- No clip embolizations occurred
- Measures of efficacy remained durable through 24 months of follow-up, and 78% of patients remained free from mitral-valve surgery

Data from Feldman T, Foster E, Glower DG, et al. Percutaneous repair or surgery for mitral regurgitation. N Engl J Med 2011;364:1395–406.

Summary

Both percutaneous and surgical groups achieved substantial clinical improvements. At 1 year, 98%

of the MitraClip patients and 88% of the surgical patients were NYHA Class I/II. Both groups had significant reductions in left ventricular (LV) and end-diastolic and end-systolic volumes and dimensions. Quality-of-life improvements were seen in both groups at 12 months, yet surgery was associated with a transient decrease in quality of life at 30 days.

The safety data from EVEREST II supported that of EVEREST I, which showed that there was a remarkably low incidence of serious adverse events with the MitraClip. In EVEREST II, the major adverse event rates at 30 days were 48% in the surgical repair group versus in 15% in the percutaneous repair group (P = .001) in an intent-to-treat analysis. The primary end point was driven by the need for more than 3 times the amount of blood transfusions in the surgical group compared with the percutaneous repair group (45% vs 13%, P<.001).

EVEREST II was the first randomized trial to compare a catheter-based MR therapy with surgical intervention. This landmark study clearly showed that despite the more profound reduction in MR severity in the surgical group versus the percutaneous group, patients who underwent percutaneous repair had significantly reduced LV end-diastolic dimensions, improved NYHA grade, and improved quality of life compared with baseline and benefited from the superior safety profile of the catheter-based approach.

Several potential explanations exist for why MitraClip recipients derived significant clinical benefit in EVEREST II despite lesser reductions in MR compared with surgery. The absolute degree of MR reduction seems to be less important than reducing the regurgitation below a critical threshold where ventricular remodeling and symptom improvement occurs. The MitraClip is clearly effective in reducing the MR below this critical threshold, accounting for the clinical improvements despite higher degrees of residual MR compared with surgery.

In addition, the echo estimates of post-MitraClip MR may have been overestimated in EVEREST II. There is a significant effect of a double orifice on the echo assessment of MR grade. The same volume of MR through a double orifice can appear to have a much greater MR area than the same volume through a single orifice, even when the area of the single-orifice and double-orifice valves are equal. This phenomenon has been well demonstrated in in vitro models.[13]

Perhaps the most striking feature of EVEREST II was the substantial difference in safety outcomes between MitraClip therapy and surgery. The safety end point was driven by a more than threefold increase in blood transfusion by more than 2 units in the surgical arm.

There is a clear mortality penalty associated with blood transfusions after open-heart operations. Patients who receive transfusions after cardiac surgery have a clearly higher mortality rate beyond 5 years postoperatively compared with patients who do not receive transfusions.[14] The risks are correlated with the number of units of blood transfused, and persist after propensity adjustment with a relative risk greater than 1.7.[15-20] Although the operative community may argue that blood transfusions should not be counted as adverse events, it is clear from the surgical literature that transfusions are not benign. The increased incidence of blood loss requiring transfusion and prolonged mechanical ventilation in the surgical group underscores decreased patient tolerance of an open thoracotomy versus a venous puncture.

The most recent data from the EVEREST trials have provided insight into patient populations who may benefit most from the MitraClip device. Subgroup analysis of EVEREST II showed the best outcomes in patients older than 75 years, with functional rather than degenerative MR, and with LV ejection fraction (LVEF) less than 60%.[12] In anatomically appropriate patients with functional MR and at high risk for surgical intervention, MitraClip therapy may be the most reasonable first option. A nonrandomized high-risk arm of EVEREST II, called the EVEREST II High-Risk Registry (HRR), sought to clarify the role of MitraClip for the treatment of high-risk patients.

EVEREST II high-risk registry

Patients enrolled in the EVEREST I phase I and EVEREST II randomized trials were considered acceptable candidates for mitral valve surgery. The aim of the EVEREST II (HRR) was to evaluate the MitraClip device in patients with elevated surgical risk.[21] Prespecified criteria qualifying a patient as high risk included age older than 75, LVEF less than 35%, prior chest surgery, and creatinine greater than 2.5 mg/dL. Seventy-eight patients with moderate to severe MR and an estimated surgical mortality risk of 12% or higher (measured with Society of Thoracic Surgery calculator or based on assessment by a surgeon) were enrolled. The prespecified mitral valve anatomic criteria were identical to those used in the randomized trial. Thirty-six patients who did not meet the anatomic screening criteria, based on transthoracic or transesophageal echo assessment, were used as a matched control group.

The HRR represented the most ill group of patients receiving the MitraClip in the EVEREST series. Most patients were elderly (>75 years) males with congestive heart failure and coronary artery disease. A substantial number of patients in the high-risk group had previous cardiac surgery (62%), moderate to severe renal disease (23%), chronic obstructive pulmonary disease (35%), and previous myocardial infarction (56%). Most of the patients in the registry had functional MR (59%), which was substantially higher than the proportion of patients with functional MR in the EVEREST I and EVEREST II randomized trials (approximately 20%).

Results

Results are summarized in **Box 3**. Devices were placed successfully in 96% of patients. Most patients had and a reduction in MR at discharge (83%), with all but 28.2% achieving a reduction in MR of 2+ or less. At 30 days, 6 months, and 12 months, patients with MR 2+ or less was

---

Box 3
Summary of results of EVEREST II high-risk registry

- In 96% of patients, devices placed successfully
- 83% of patients had reduction in MR at discharge
- All but 28.2% achieved a reduction in MR ≤2+
- 72.9%, 73.3%, and 77.8% of patients had MR of 2+ or less at 30 days, 6 months, and 12 months
  - statistically significant change from baseline
- At 30 days and 1 year, significant improvements seen in
  - LV dimensions
  - NYHA class
  - quality-of-life scores
- 45% decrease from baseline in annual hospitalizations for heart failure as a result of MitraClip therapy
  - these effects present in both the functional MR and degenerative MR groups
- Overall 30-day mortality in the HRR group and control groups were similar (7.7% and 8.3%, respectively)
  - significantly lower than predicted surgical mortality of 18.2% for open heart mitral valve surgery in this patient cohort (P = .006).
- At 1 year, survival was improved in the HRR group compared with the control group (76.4% vs 55.3%, P = .047).

72.9%, 73.3%, and 77.8%, respectively, which represented a statistically significant change from baseline. In the HRR, significant improvements were seen in LV dimensions, NYHA class, and quality-of-life scores at 30 days and 1 year. Annual hospitalizations for heart failure in the HRR were decreased as a result of MitraClip therapy by 45% from baseline. These beneficial effects were present in both the functional MR and degenerative MR groups.

Overall 30-day mortality in the HRR group and control groups were similar (7.7% and 8.3%, respectively) and significantly lower than predicted surgical mortality of 18.2% for open heart mitral valve surgery in this patient cohort (P = .006). At 1 year, survival was improved in the HRR group compared with the control group (76.4% vs 55.3%, P = .047).

Summary

The high-risk patient population included in EVEREST HRR represents a group that has never been treated with surgery in the past or has never been included in surgical registries. These generally older, poorly functioning patients have poor prognosis and limited therapeutic options. The favorable effect of MitraClip therapy on the LV dimensions, clinical heart failure symptoms, and quality-of-life parameters in these patients is striking. The results of the HRR are largely consistent with the European experience for patient selection since commercialization of the device there in 2008, where a large proportion of patients who, undergoing the MitraClip procedure, have functional MR, are at high risk for surgery, and have derived significant anatomic and functional benefits from this technology.[22]

REALISM

The REALISM continued access registry was created to continue to offer MitraClip therapy to select patients when the EVEREST II trial completed enrollment in September 2008. REALISM is a prospective, multicenter, continued-access registry of the EVEREST II study. Patients with moderate to severe MR are currently being enrolled at 38 centers in the United States. There are 2 groups to which patients are assigned: a high-risk arm and non–high-risk arm. Clinical follow-up data are collected at 30 days, 6 months, and 12 months. There is an emphasis on the assessment of quality of life and functional capacity following MitraClip therapy. To date, the registry has primarily enrolled elderly patients with functional MR who tend to be high risk for mitral valve surgery. This pattern of patient selection is consistent with the subgroup analysis in EVEREST II, and also with the use of

MitraClip in the European experience since it became commercially available in 2008.[22]

LIMITATIONS OF THE MITRACLIP DEVICE

Despite its obvious potential, there are several recognized limitations to the MitraClip therapy. The device requires introduction of a 24-Fr guide catheter to the femoral vein, which has potential to cause vascular damage and injury of the intra-atrial septum. Despite this, blood transfusions continued to be far more prevalent in the surgical arm of the randomized trial. The septum seems to heal in the vast majority of patients and atrial septal defect has not been a significant problem in the trial experience to date. Delivery of the implantable clip is technically demanding, and requires extensive training. This was evident in the feasibility registry, where procedure times in the first third of the cohort were an hour longer than in the final third of the cohort, even when performed by interventionalists with extensive experience in catheter-based procedures. New sites that have started using this device commercially in Europe have benefited from the prior experience, and the learning curve has been shortened with the accumulation of shared experience.

The long-term durability of MR reduction is unknown. Clinical data beyond 3 years of follow-up are not yet available after MitraClip treatment. The surgical experience with isolated edge-to-edge repair has shown durable results to 12 years.[23]

There is some concern that the chance for mitral surgery may be lost after placement of a MitraClip. Patients have undergone successful repair as long as 5 years after placement of a clip. It is clear that in some cases repair may not be possible after a MitraClip procedure. It appears that many of the valve replacements have been in patients at higher risk for failed repair, such as those with anterior or bi-leaflet prolapse, or with calcified mitral annulus. It is important that a surgeon who intends to remove a MitraClip understands how to unlock the device, to avoid damage to the leaflets.[24]

The MitraClip device is not applicable to all subsets of patients with MR, particularly those with rheumatic disease, annular calcification involving the grasping area of the leaflets, or ruptured papillary muscles. Patients must meet specific anatomic criteria to be considered for the device, and many potential candidates are turned down because of inappropriate mitral valve anatomy. Additionally, concerns have been raised by the surgical community that percutaneous edge-to-edge repair alone, despite its demonstrated ability to improve LV dimensions, may not be sufficient to fully prevent annular dilatation in functional MR. As is the case for surgical annuloplasty for functional MR, the primary problem for many patients is LV dysfunction, which is not remedied by conventional mitral repair.

Percutaneous annuloplasty devices that address progressive annular dilatation are in phase I trials, and may eventually be used alone or in combination with the MitraClip to address annular dilation. As more novel percutaneous therapies become available, a wider range of patients will be considered candidates for percutaneous management of MR.

SUMMARY

In the randomized EVEREST II trial, 80% of patients were free of need for surgery 1 year after MitraClip therapy. Although percutaneous repair was less effective at reducing MR than conventional surgery, the procedure was associated with superior safety and similar improvements in clinical outcomes. The US EVEREST trial experience, in combination with the commercial use of the MitraClip device in Europe, has enabled more than 3000 patients to benefit from this novel therapy. It is clear that the MitraClip offers significant clinical and quality-of-life benefit to patients, with an excellent safety profile compared with surgical intervention. The patient population that benefits most from this therapy appears to be older, high-risk or inoperable patients with functional or degenerative MR, who otherwise have limited or no therapeutic options.

REFERENCES

1. Fedak P, McCarthy P, Bonow R. Evolving concepts and technologies in mitral valve repair. Circulation 2008;117(7):963–74.
2. Alfieri O, Maisano F, De Bonis B, et al. The double-orifice technique in mitral valve repair: a simple solution for complex problems. J Thorac Cardiovasc Surg 2001;122:674–81.
3. Alfieri O, De Bonis M. The role of the edge-to-edge repair in the surgical treatment of mitral regurgitation. J Card Surg 2010;25:536–41.
4. St. Goar FG, Fann JI, Komtebedde J, et al. Endovascular edge-to-edge mitral valve repair: acute results in a porcine model. Circulation 2003;108:1990–3.
5. Fann J, St. Goar F, Komtebedde J, et al. Off pump edge-to-edge mitral valve technique using a mechanical clip in a chronic model. Circulation 2003;108:17: IV–493.
6. Fann JI, St. Goar FG, Komtebedde J, et al. Beating heart catheter-based edge-to-edge mitral valve

procedure in a porcine model: efficacy and healing response. Circulation 2004;110:988–93.

7. Ladich E, Michaels MB, Jones RM, et al, on behalf of the EVEREST Investigators. The pathologic healing response of explanted MitraClip devices. Circulation 2011;123:1418–27.

8. Condado JA, Acquatella H, Rodriguez L, et al. Percutaneous edge-to-edge mitral valve repair: 2-year follow-up in the first human case. Catheter Cardiovasc Interv 2006;67:323–5.

9. Feldman T, Wasserman HS, Herrmann HC, et al. Percutaneous mitral valve repair using the edge-to-edge technique: six-month results of the Everest phase I clinical trial. J Am Coll Cardiol 2005;46:2134–40.

10. Bonow RO, Carabello BA, Chatterjee K, et al. 2008 focused update incorporated into the ACC/AHA 2006 guidelines for the management of patients with valvular heart disease: a report of the American College of Cardiology/American Heart Association Task Force on Practice Guidelines (Writing Committee to Develop Guidelines for the Management of Patients With Valvular Heart Disease). J Am Coll Cardiol 2008;52:e1–142.

11. Mauri L, Garg P, Massaro JM, et al. The Everest II trial: design and rationale for a randomized study of the evalve mitraclip system compared with mitral valve surgery for mitral regurgitation. Am Heart J 2010;160:23–9.

12. Feldman T, Foster E, Glower DG, et al. Percutaneous repair or surgery for mitral regurgitation. N Engl J Med 2011;364:1395–406.

13. Lin BA, Forouhar AS, Pahlevan NM, et al. Color Doppler jet area overestimates regurgitant column when multiple jets are present. J Am Soc Echocardiogr 2010;23(9):993–1000.

14. Murphy GJ, Reeves BC, Rogers CA, et al. Increased mortality, postoperative morbidity, and cost after red blood cell transfusion in patients having cardiac surgery. Circulation 2007;116:2544–52.

15. Engoren MC, Habib RH, Zacharias A, et al. Effect of blood transfusion on long-term survival after cardiac operation. Ann Thorac Surg 2002;74:1180–6.

16. Koch CG, Li L, Duncan AI, et al. Morbidity and mortality risk associated with red blood cell and blood-component transfusion in isolated coronary artery bypass grafting. Crit Care Med 2006;34:1608–16.

17. Koch CG, Li L, Duncan AI, et al. Transfusion in coronary artery bypass grafting is associated with reduced long-term survival. Ann Thorac Surg 2006;81:1650–7.

18. Kuduvalli M, Oo AY, Newall N, et al. Effect of perioperative red blood cell transfusion on 30-day and 1-year mortality following coronary artery bypass surgery. Eur J Cardiothorac Surg 2005;27:592–8.

19. Scott BH, Seifert FC, Grimson R. Blood transfusion is associated with increased resource utilisation, morbidity and mortality in cardiac surgery. Ann Card Anaesth 2008;11:15–9.

20. Surgenor SD, DeFoe GR, Fillinger MP, et al. Intraoperative red blood cell transfusion during coronary artery bypass graft surgery increases the risk of postoperative low-output heart failure. Circulation 2006;114:I43–8.

21. Whitlow PL, Feldman T, Pederson W, et al. The EVEREST II high risk study: acute and 12 month results with catheter based mitral leaflet repair, in press.

22. Franzen O, Baldus S, Rudolph V, et al. Acute outcomes of mitraclip therapy for mitral regurgitation in high-surgical-risk patients: emphasis on adverse valve morphology and severe left ventricular dysfunction. Eur Heart J 2010;31:1373–81.

23. Maisano F, Vigano G, Blasio A, et al. Surgical isolated edge-to-edge mitral repair without annuloplasty: clinical proof of principle for an endovascular approach. EuroIntervention 2006;2:181–6.

24. Argenziano M, Skipper, Heimansohn D. Surgical revision after percutaneous mitral repair with the MitraClip device. Ann Thorac Surg 2010;89:72–80.

Percutaneous Treatment of Primary and Secondary Mitral Regurgitation: Overall Scope of the Problem

Chad Kliger, MD, Carlos E. Ruiz, MD, PhD, FSCAI*

KEYWORDS

- Mitral Regurgitation • Primary regurgitation
- Secondary regurgitation • Percutaneous treatment

Mitral regurgitation (MR) is a heterogeneous disorder requiring the understanding of complex mitral anatomy and pathophysiology. Advanced imaging has furthered our knowledge and ability to treat patients with this disorder. With the increasing population of MR, patients not referred for surgery, and the desire for less-invasive treatment approaches, a multitude of percutaneous options have emerged. This review is written for interventionalists to fully appreciate the overall scope of mitral regurgitation. Understanding and integrating mitral anatomy with pathophysiology, multimodality imaging, and current transcatheter mitral therapies are paramount for treating this disorder.

ANATOMY OF MITRAL REGURGITATION

The mitral valve (MV) apparatus is a complex structure that requires the functional integrity of 6 anatomic components (**Box 1**). These components include the left atrioventricular junction (LAVJ) or annulus, the mitral leaflets or cusps, the chordae tendinae, the papillary muscles, the left ventricular (LV) wall and the posterior left atrial (LA) wall.[1] LV systole initiates with contraction of ventricular myocardium along with its papillary muscles. The resultant vertical forces move the mitral leaflets into apposition. The rise in LV pressure initiates coaptation of the leaflet-free edges, with the remainder of the leaflets parachuting

into the LA. The annulus is the fulcrum for the leaflets and with ventricular systole, decreases in size to allow for ease of coaptation.[2,3] The surface area of the leaflets is approximately 2.5 times the area of the orifice. During ejection, the apex and mitral orifice approach each other along with papillary muscle contraction applying the appropriate force to the chordae tendinae, preventing eversion of the leaflets. For normal closure of the MV, both leaflets must align in the same plane as they coapt, requiring an optimal annular size, a geometrically correct orientation of the papillary muscles giving rise to the tendinous cords, and appropriate closing forces generated by LV muscular contraction.[4] For MR to occur, at least one of the mitral apparatus components must have fault.

Left Atrioventricular Junction

LAVJ, also referred to as the mitral annulus, is the D-shaped orifice or hinge line formed at the convergence of the LA walls and the supporting LV structures.[4,7] The LAVJ is hyperbolic paraboloid (saddle-shaped) in appearance with elevated septal and lateral segments and a complementary depressed medial segment along the central zone of apposition.[8] Along the depressed anterior segment of the LAVJ, the anterior mitral leaflet is in fibrous continuity with both the noncoronary

Lenox Hill Heart and Vascular Institute, Department of Cardiovascular Disease, Division of Structural and Congenital Heart Disease, 130 East 77th Street, 9th Floor Black Hall Building, New York, NY 10075, USA
* Corresponding author.
E-mail address: CRuiz@NSHS.edu

Intervent Cardiol Clin 1 (2012) 73–83
doi:10.1016/j.iccl.2011.09.009

and left coronary leaflets of the aortic valve, described as the aortic-mitral curtain. On either side of the aortic-mitral curtain is fibrous tissue, called the left and right fibrous trigones, which connects the anterior leaflet to the ventricular myocardium. The right trigone is continuous with the membranous ventricular septum and is the site of the atrioventricular (AV) node. The depressed posterior segment of the LAVJ merges with the musculature of the LV inflow and the base of the posterior mitral leaflet.

The saddle-shaped appearance of the LAVJ helps reduce mechanical stress on the leaflets. During systole, the mitral annulus contracts, reducing the area that the opposing leaflets need to coapt by an estimated 20% to 50%.[3] LV dilation may distend the mitral annulus, reducing the ability for the annulus to contract.[2] A loss in systolic annular contraction, also noted in calcification of the annulus, can lead to leaflet malapposition.[9]

Mitral Leaflets

The MV is bifoliate, consisting of the anterior (aortic) leaflet in fibrous continuity with the aortic valve and the opposing posterior (mural) leaflet.[7] The leaflets are made of connective tissue intertwined with striated muscle, enveloped by endocardial cells. The striated muscle fibers are in direct continuity with the LA muscle, helping to promote closure of the MV.[10] The areas of the 2 leaflets are identical. Given the shorter base of the anterior leaflet, however, the length from the free margin to the annulus is 2 or more times that of the posterior leaflet.[1] The base of the posterior leaflet, in contrast, occupies two-thirds of the annular circumference. The anterior leaflet tends to be more mobile whereas the posterior leaflet acts as a support structure.[11] Both leaflets are a single continuous structure that becomes confluent at the commissures. There are multiple scallops separated by slits in the posterior leaflet

only (P1, P2, and P3), to accommodate the curved shape of the closure line. No scallops are present in the anterior leaflet to avoid LV outflow tract obstruction. The closure line or zone of apposition between the leaflets is obliquely oriented relative to the orthogonal planes of the body, inferoseptally and superolaterally. Leaflet abnormalities generally include excessive or deficient leaflet tissue or restricted mobility.

Chordae Tendinae

The MV leaflets are attached to the LV wall via the chordae tendinae (tendinous cords) and the papillary muscles. The chordae tendinae are avascular structures composed of an undulated pattern of collagen fibrils covered by a dense layer of elastic fibers.[12] This framework establishes its strong physical properties of elasticity, strength, and endurance. The chordae originate from the papillary muscles and attach to the free edges and the ventricular side of the mitral leaflets.[4] They transmit contractions from the papillary muscles to the valve leaflets. The fibrils straighten when stretched by papillary muscle contraction; on relaxation, the elastic tissue returns the collagen to its inherent wavy configuration.

There are 3 types of chordae: primary or marginal, secondary, and tertiary or basal.[7] The primary chordae enter the leaflet in their free margin or rough zone. The secondary chordae enter in the region beyond the free margin called the clear zone. Each papillary muscle distributes primary and secondary chords to the ipsilateral half of both leaflets. They maintain leaflet apposition and facilitate valve closure. The tertiary chordae originate directly from the ventricular wall, not the papillary muscles, and attach exclusively to the ventricular surface of the posterior leaflet. They are important in maintaining ventricular geometry and the support for the LAVJ. The thicker and longer secondary chordae, called the strut chords, insert into the undersurface of the anterior leaflet and constitute the interface between the LV myocardium and the annulus at the fibrous trigones.[4] This anatomic junction is termed the papillary-annular continuity. The anterior strut chords provide the translational mechanics of the leaflet, more anteriorly, rendering a funnel-shaped mitral inflow facilitating blood into the LV during diastole.

Abnormalities of the chordae tendinae include abnormally long or short chordae, ectopically inserted chordae, and ruptured chordae.[1] The undulating pattern of collagen fibers gradually changes with age by elongation of the waves and also thinning of the cross-sectional area. The chordae are also the thinnest at their insertion site on the leaflets, the most common site of rupture. Transection of the secondary chordae does not cause mitral regurgitation. The lack of strut chords at the papillary-annular continuity can predispose to annular dilatation and calcification, precluding poor leaflet coaptation. Furthermore, transection of the strut chords disrupts normal axial blood flow in the mitral orifice and LV outflow tract, and transection of the tertiary chordae disrupts ventricular geometry and LAVJ support.

Papillary Muscles

The chordae tendinae, except the tertiary chordae, arise from paired papillary muscles and extend to both mitral leaflets. There are 2 papillary muscles, the superolateral (anterolateral) and the inferoseptal (posteromedial), both originating from the apical to middle thirds of the LV free wall.[11] During diastole, the papillary muscles do not protrude into the submitral space to facilitate mitral inflow. During systole, however, they bulge into the LV cavity, redirecting flow toward the aortic valve, forming part of the LV outflow tract. The superolateral papillary muscle is supplied by one or more branches of the left circumflex artery or diagonal branches of the left anterior descending artery. The inferoseptal papillary muscle, however, is supplied by a single branch of the left circumflex artery or right coronary artery, depending on vessel dominance. Given its singular vascular supply, the inferoseptal papillary muscle is more susceptible to coronary ischemia and complications. Papillary dysfunction can occur either with rupture through infarction or trauma (generally leading to sudden death) or with fibrosis or ischemia. As the LV apex moves toward the annulus during systole, the chordae provide slack, allowing the leaflets to prolapse into the LA. Elongated degenerated papillary muscles can induce prolapse and retracted papillary muscles can make cords vulnerable to rupture. Papillary muscle rupture results in acute loss of leaflet support and subsequent MR with the location of rupture associated with the degree of regurgitation and clinical outcomes.

Left Ventricular and Left Atrial Walls

The LV and LA walls also play an important role in MV integrity. The papillary muscles and the LV wall represent the muscular components of the mitral apparatus. The direction of tension on the leaflets by the papillary muscles is in a vertical orientation to the mitral annulus. When LV dilatation occurs, the papillary muscles are displaced laterally due to the spherical shape of the ventricle. The position of the papillary muscles and their direction of tension on the leaflets change from vertical to lateral as well. Lateral tension, especially on the anterior leaflet, opposes leaflet apposition. More pronounced dilatation could displace the papillary muscles in an apical direction, not allowing for leaflet coaptation. Furthermore, the LA and LV support the posterior leaflet of the MV. The inferolateral wall of the LV directly supports the posterior leaflet through the tertiary chordae tendinae. LV dilatation or dyskinesis can alter the orientation of the tertiary cords and tether the posterior leaflet. The LA walls have continuity to the mitral apparatus through the fibrous trigones and aortic-mitral curtain to the anterior mitral leaflet. Dilatation of the LA can displace its posterior wall, posteriorly and downward.[1,13] Due to its support in the aortic-mitral curtain, posterior atrial wall displacement places tension on the posterior leaflet and causes MR.

Related Coronary Artery and Venous Structures

The great cardiac vein, also known as the anterior interventricular vein, originates in the anterior interventricular groove alongside the left anterior descending artery.[14,15] It courses toward the base of the heart and then directs inferiorly in the AV groove. The great cardiac vein merges with the oblique vein of the LA becoming the coronary sinus. The middle cardiac vein courses along the inferior interventricular groove and empties into the coronary sinus near its ostium. The caliber of the coronary sinus increases closer to its ostium. The course of the coronary sinus is variable.[16] Predominately, the body of the sinus is adjacent to the inferior wall of the LA, superior and cranial to the LAVJ.[4] It is closest to the lateral segment of the LAVJ at the midpoint of the posterior leaflet and farthest away at the endpoint of the line of leaflet apposition. With the presence of significant mitral regurgitation, the posterior segment portion of the coronary sinus elevates superiorly and cranially closer to the endpoints, coinciding with an increase in the septal-lateral annular diameter and flattening of the mitral annulus.[17] Adjacent to the coronary sinus is the left circumflex artery, intersecting the coronary sinus in a majority of patients, but with a variable course. In rare cases, the coronary sinus can cross diagonal and ramus branch arteries.

PATHOPHYSIOLOGY OF MITRAL REGURGITATION: PRIMARY AND SECONDARY

A fault in any of the anatomic components of the mitral apparatus leads to mitral regurgitation. Either alone or in combination, abnormalities are caused by a particular pathophysiologic process that helps further categorize this disorder and consider options for mechanical correction. MR can be divided into primary (organic) and secondary (functional) MR. In primary MR, there are inherent problems with the mitral apparatus. This category can be further divided into congenital and degenerative MR (**Fig. 1**). Conversely, in secondary MR, the mitral apparatus itself is usually normal. Secondary MR is a result of geometric and/or functional changes of the LV/LA that indirectly alters the mitral apparatus. This can be further divided into ischemic and myocardial-cell dysfunction (nonischemic). It is the complex interaction of anatomic abnormalities with geometric and functional factors that define this disease.

Primary MR is an anatomic problem with the valve apparatus that can only be corrected with an anatomic solution, restoration of valve competence.[18] Secondary MR, alternatively, is a mechanical problem either through an ischemic or nonischemic cardiomyopathy that has caused an anatomically normal valve to become regurgitant. Despite correction of MR, the underlying mechanical abnormality will still exist. Unlike primary MR, secondary MR is a cause for worsened prognosis.[19,20] Determining if it is

a reasonable target for intervention or which patient population may benefit has yet to be determined.

As recently published, a modified classification of percutaneous MV repair options, categorized according to functional anatomy and device action, aids in tailoring device therapies for the different types of MR.[21] **Table 1** helps interventionalists categorize MR patients by integrating pathophysiology and anatomic abnormalities to the type of MR and the current devices available. As the technology improves, so does the application of these technologies and the possibilities for combining techniques to improve procedural success. The remainder of the discussion focuses on MV imaging and the active available technologies for percutaneous MV intervention.

IMAGING IN MITRAL REGURGITATION

Evaluation of the underlying mechanism of MR and determining the presence of suitable valve and LV anatomy and geometry are crucial in the assessment and planning for transcatheter therapy (**Box 2**). Furthermore, understanding MV function both before and during MV intervention help in selection of appropriate device therapies and

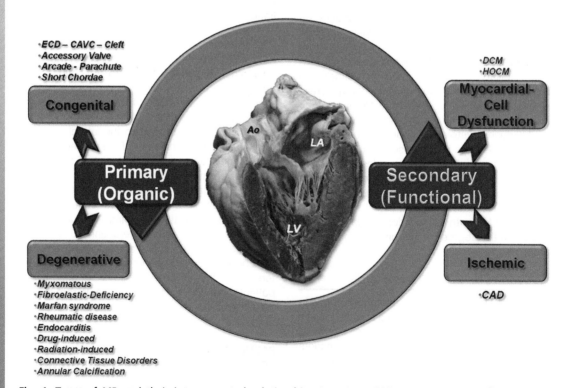

Fig. 1. Types of MR and their interconnected relationship. Ao, aorta; CAD, coronary artery disease; CAVC, complete antrioventricular canal defect; DCM, dilated cardiomyopathy; ECD, endocardial cushion defect; HOCM, hypertrophic cardiomyopathy.

Table 1
The anatomic fault of the mitral apparatus with its associated focus of treatment, type of MR treated, and current devices available

Anatomic Fault	Focus of Treatment	Category of MR Treated	Devices Available
LAVJ (mitral annulus)	Decrease circumference of the valvular orifice	Secondary	Indirect annuloplasty via CS: Carillon Direct annuloplasty via mechanical: Mitralign, enCorSQ, Millipede, Cardinal, Cardioban Direct annuloplasty via energy mediated: QuantumCor, ReCor
Mitral leaflets	Decrease size of mitral orifice by bringing leaflets together or restricting leaflet mobility	Primary and secondary	Leaflet plication: MitraClip (primary and some secondary MR) Leaflet ablation: Thermocool (primary MR) Leaflet coaptation: Percu-Pro (secondary MR)
Chordae tendinae	Restoration of chordal function	Primary	Artificial chordal implants: NeoChord, MitraFlex, V-Chordal
LV dilation	Decrease the anterior-posterior dimensions of the LV	Secondary	LV remodeling: iCoapsys
Mitral leaflets and chordae tendinae	Decrease circumference of the valvular orifice and restore chordal function	Primary	Leaflet plication and chordal implants: MitraFlex

Box 2
Comparison of imaging modalities for mitral regurgitation

3-D transesophageal echocardiography (TEE)

- Provides accurate real-time images
- Permits visualization in multiple orientations, allowing for the localization of the largest regurgitant orifice and more accurate characterization of MR mechanism than 2-D echocardiography
- Can provide complementary information on the valvular structure and function before, during, and immediately after MV procedures

Multidetector row CT (MDCT)

- Provides 3-D acquisition of the entire heart throughout the cardiac cycle
- Enables the construction of images in multiple planes via multiplanar reformation
- Evaluates the coronary arteries, accurately differentiates primary from secondary MR compared with TTE
- Identifies all causes of chronic MR, especially in complex cases where more than one cause may be present
- Enables accurate 3-D visualization of the mitral leaflets
- Can provide useful information on the dimensions of the coronary sinus and its position relative to the mitral annulus and coronary arteries
- Provides accurate characterization of the LV dimensions, anatomy and location of the papillary muscles and location, and extent of MV apparatus calcification[5,6]
- Can determine potential interference with the papillary muscles and coronary arteries during implantation of LV remodeling devices

guide procedures to optimize device performance. Historically, 2-D echocardiography has been the most common modality used to assess valvular heart disease. Because of the complex configuration of the MV apparatus, however, 2-D imaging techniques are limited.[22] With the recent advent of 3-D TEE, understanding of MV anatomy and geometry and its relationships to other cardiac structures has grown significantly.[23,24] 3-D TEE provides accurate real-time images and permits visualization in multiple orientations, allowing for the localization of the largest regurgitant orifice and more accurate characterization of MR mechanism than 2-D echocardiography.[25] Being able to offer superior accuracy to assess MR has furthered the ability to understand its complexities.[26]

Multidetector row computed tomography (MDCT) provides another way of accurately assessing the anatomy, geometry, and spatial relationships of the MV apparatus.[5] MDCT provides 3-D acquisition of the entire heart throughout the cardiac cycle and enables the construction of images in multiple planes via multiplanar reformation. CT data reconstructed in smaller increments, 5% throughout the R-R interval, maintain a high spatial resolution with improved temporal resolution. This also enables identification of the systolic frame where failure of mitral leaflet coaptation occurs. With its ability to evaluate the coronary arteries, MDCT can accurately differentiate primary from secondary MR compared with TTE and identify all causes of chronic MR, especially complex cases where more than one may be present.

MDCT enables accurate 3-D visualization of the mitral leaflets and can provide useful information on the dimensions of the coronary sinus and its position relative to the mitral annulus and coronary arteries.[14,16] MDCT also provides accurate characterization of the LV dimensions, anatomy, and location of the papillary muscles and location and extent of MV apparatus calcification.[5,6] It can determine the potential interference with the papillary muscles and coronary arteries during implantation of LV remodeling devices. For the most part, combining the axial views and 3-D volume renderings, feasibility and safety of many of the devices can be anticipated during preprocedural screening by visualizing the position of the device along with important related cardiac structures.[27]

3-D TEE can provide complementary information on the valvular structure and function before, during, and immediately after MV procedures.[28,29] The knowledge obtained from both modalities, 3-D TEE, and MDCT can permit accurate procedural planning and may result in a significant shortening of fluoroscopy and procedural times. Overall, the combination of 3-D TEE and MDCT may provide the most accurate information to help select candidates for specific transcatheter therapies, and the combination of fluoroscopy and intraprocedural 2-D/3-D TEE may provide the real-time feedback necessary for procedural guidance.[30] A multidisciplinary imaging approach to MR will help maximize procedural success and reduce therapeutic-related complications.

DISORDERS OF THE LEFT ATRIOVENTRICULAR JUNCTION

The goal of annuloplasty when the LAVJ is dilated is to decrease the circumference of the valvular orifice, reducing the septal-lateral diameter by at least 8 mm. Annuloplasty techniques are designed to restore annular size and shape, thus improving leaflet coaptation. This is accomplished while preserving the patency of the coronary sinus and left circumflex arteries, reducing damage to the AV node, and preserving the anatomic relation of the LAVJ. A majority of these devices are used for patients with functional MR, where changes in mitral annular geometry play an important role. Indirect options for correction include reshaping or restraining the valvular orifice via the coronary sinus. Direct options for correction include intracardiac reshaping or restraining via the LA or LV.

Indirect Annuloplasty: Via Coronary Sinus

Indirect annuloplasty uses the coronary sinus (CS) to reshape the valvular orifice based on the close proximity of the CS to the MV. This approach redirects the posterior annulus anteriorly, decreasing the septal-lateral dimension and improving leaflet coaptation. The difficulty with this technique is that the CS only relates to the posterior portion of the annulus (half the perimeter of the mitral annulus) and that there is variability in the CS anatomy. In many cases, the CS does not course in the AV groove along the left AV junction. The increased distance from the CS to the mitral annulus, called atrialization, worsens in severe MR with annular dilatation. Device deployment may then be suboptimal for improving valvular dynamics. Furthermore, the CS may directly transverse the coronary arteries. The diagonal or ramus arteries cross between the CS and mitral annulus in approximately 16% of patients and the left circumflex artery artery in 60% to 80% of patients.[14–16] Anatomic evaluation to assess the relationship of the coronary arteries to the CS and mitral annulus is necessary before indirect annuloplasty.

Other considerations that would limit the use of these devices include mitral annular calcification that make it difficult to reshape the annulus, the presence of CS pacing leads that would make implantation impossible, and small coronary venous system increasing the potential for perforations.[21,31] Placement of indirect annuloplasty devices may also prevent the future placement of CS leads for cardiac resynchronization. Early reports of cardiac vein access after annuloplasty, however, show potential.[31] Devices are usually delivered via internal jugular or subclavian venous access, because the CS ostium is at the base of the right atrium.

The Carillon Mitral Contour System (Cardiac Dimensions, Kirkland, WA, USA) is a double anchor device with a fixed-length nitinol bridge between nitinol wire anchors. The proximal anchor is deployed in the anterior interventricular vein and the distal anchor in the great cardiac vein. After the distal anchor is deployed, the bridge is unsheathed, and tension is applied to the bridge. Anterior displacement of the posterior annulus and degree of MR can be assessed immediately via echocardiography or ventriculography and tension on the bridge can be adjusted to achieve optimal results. Once the desired effect is achieved, the proximal anchor is deployed. The device can be retrieved if a nonoptimal result is achieved. In the Carillon Mitral Annuloplasty Device European Union Study (AMADEUS) and Tighten the Annulus Now (TITAN) trials, successful device implantation was demonstrated in 62% of patients with a mean grade reduction of MR of 1.[32,33] More than one-third of the patients had insufficient reduction in MR or coronary artery compression that prevented use.

Direct Annuloplasty

Direct annuloplasty directly reshapes the mitral annulus, without using the CS. Devices are delivered into either the LA or the LV and implanted directly into the mitral annulus. Heat energy can also be applied to alter the size of the mitral annulus. These technologies may reduce the potential complications noted by the CS approach and may have an application for patients with secondary MR, as well as in degenerative MR.

Mechanical Approach

The Mitralign device (Tewksbury, MA, USA) is delivered retrograde into the LV into the periannular space. Anchors are deployed on the posterior mitral annulus at P1/P2 and P2/P3 locations, connected by a suture. Tension is placed on the suture, cinching the device and in turn the mitral

annulus.[34] Procedural success has been noted in 86% of the patients.[35] The Accucinch Annuloplasty system (Guided Delivery Systems, Santa Clara, CA, USA) uses a similar technique as the Mitralign device. The device, however, is delivered via a transapical approach with the placement of up to 12 anchors applied from P1 to P3, extending from the right trigone to left trigone. A suture connects the anchors with direct tension placed on the suture that decreases posterior annular size. Early enrollment in to CINCH2 trial revealed procedural success with significant reductions in MR.

The major limitation of these devices is that they are partial rings, cinching the posterior mitral annulus only. Placement of a complete mitral annuloplasty band/rings is currently being evaluated, enCorSQ (MiCardia, Irving, CA, USA), Millipede (Ann Arbor, MI, USA), Cardinal and Cardioban (Valtech Cardio, Or-Yehuda, Israel) systems. Complete annuloplasty rings were initially placed via minimally invasive approach, but now transseptal or retrograde systems are being developed. These rings are fixed into the periannular space, adjustable for appropriate MR result by echocardiography. Clinical safety and feasibility is still pending.

Energy-Mediated Approach

Direct annuloplasty using an energy-mediated approach occurs by applying heat energy, either through radiofrequency (RF) energy or high-intensity focused ultrasound, to the mitral annulus. Heat energy causes thermal remodeling of the annular collagen resulting in scarring and a reduction in the annular size. The QuantumCor (Lake Forest, CA, USA) and ReCor (Paris, France) systems use RF and high-intensity focused ultrasound energy, respectively, and are undergoing safety and feasibility evaluation.[36] The concern for overscarring of the mitral annulus due to their lack of precision application may lead to resultant mitral stenosis. Damage or perforation of surrounding cardiac structures is possible and remains a concern with these devices.

DISORDERS OF MITRAL LEAFLETS
Leaflet Plication

Percutaneous leaflet plication decreases the size of the mitral orifice by application of a suture, which brings the anterior and posterior leaflets (A2 and P2 segments) together, creating an effective double-orifice MV. This technique, based on the surgical Alfieri technique, re-establishes leaflet coaptation and subsequently reduces mitral regurgitation.[37] Leaflet plication restores leaflet coaptation but does not address the annular component of mitral regurgitation. The Alfieri technique without annuloplasty has been shown less effective and more frequently required reoperation due to MR recurrence.[38,39] Nonetheless, a select group of patients who have undergone surgical isolated edge-to-edge repair without annuloplasty have demonstrated clinical benefit.

The MitraClip system (Abbott Vascular, Abbott Park, IL, USA) uses a steerable catheter (24F proximally and 22F distally) to deliver a metallic clip to the LV via a transseptal approach, allowing grasping of the free edges of the mitral leaflets.[28] The anatomic requirements to accommodate this approach include a centrally located MR jet associated with the A2-P2 segments, a sufficient length of coaptation of at least 2 mm, a coaptation depth (the displacement of the leaflets from the mitral annulus) of less than 11 mm, and if involving a flail mitral leaflet, a flail gap and flail width not exceeding 10 mm and 15 mm, respectively. The MitraClip can be repositioned or removed before deployment and multiple clips can be implanted to achieve the desired MR reduction. This technique has demonstrated a significant reduction in MR in patients primarily with primary degenerative MR, with some role in secondary MR.

The Endovascular Valve Edge-to-Edge Repair Study (EVEREST) evaluated the safety and feasibility of the MitraClip system.[40] Procedural success was achieved in 74% of patients (n = 107) with a resultant reduction in MR to less than 2+. One clip was used in 65 patients (61%), 2 clips in 31 patients (29%), and in the remaining 19 patients (10%) the clip was not implanted due to failure to reduce MR or transseptal complications. Partial clip detachment occurred in less than 10% of cases, with no clip embolizations or procedural-related mortality. Of the patients with procedural success, 3-year survival rate was 90.1% with a 76.3% freedom from surgery. In those requiring surgery, surgical options were preserved with 84% undergoing MV repair.[41]

The EVEREST II study (n = 279) evaluated the MitraClip system further when compared with conventional MV surgery.[42] Patients were randomized in a 2:1 fashion to either MitraClip or surgery. Successful reduction in MR by at least 1 grade was achieved in 76% of MitraClip patients. Composite endpoints of freedom from death, MV surgery, or reoperation more than 90 days after procedure and MR greater than 2+ at 1 year were 72.4% and 87.8% (MitraClip and surgery, respectively, noninferior). The MitraClip was associated with a significant improvement in NYHA class compared with surgery with superiority in safety endpoints, including blood transfusion greater than 2 units (9.5% vs 57%). Seventy-nine percent of patients had degenerative MR and 21% had secondary MR. Similar results were achieved regardless of the MR type and were maintained at 3 years.

Ablation

Leaflet ablation occurs by the application of RF energy to the anterior leaflet and its associated chordae, effectively heating the local tissue causing fibrotic scarring.[43,44] Structural and functional alterations result from thickening and contracture of the valve leaflet and surrounding structures, leading to restricted leaflet mobility. The population treated with this technique is primary degenerative MR, predominately myxomatous MV prolapse with a weakened central fibrous core of both the leaflet and chordae, increased leaflet surface area, and increased chordae extensibility.[45–47] The Thermocool irrigation ablation catheter (Biosense Webster, Diamond Bar, CA, USA) is the RF ablation catheter available and has been evaluated in animal models. It is delivered retrograde into the LV and uses intracardiac echocardiography to assist in directed ablation. The lack of precision with the device can produce varying results with the potential for worsening of MR, leaflet perforation, or damage to nearby structures. Long-term effects on valve fragility/instability and human application have yet to be determined.

Leaflet Coaptation

Failure of the mitral leaflets to fully coapt is common, specifically in patients with functional MR but also in patients with primary degenerative MR. The Percu-Pro system (Cardiosolutions, Stoughton, MA, USA) has a polyurethane-silicone polymer balloon, also referred to as a leaflet space occupier, that positions itself within the MV orifice at the coaptation zone. The balloon is anchored to the interventricular septum or apex by a mitral spacer anchor, connected by a connection cable. The balloon floats across the exposed MV orifice providing a surface against which the leaflets can coapt, reducing mitral regurgitation. It is deployed either through the transfemoral or transapical approaches. The device does not alter the MV apparatus and is reversible. Potential complications with the system include thrombus formation on the device and iatrogenic mitral stenosis. The first human experience with the device resulted in a 1-grade to 2-grade reduction in MR without a significant transmitral gradient.[48]

DISORDERS OF THE CHORDAE TENDINAE: CHORDAL IMPLANTS

Chordal implants are synthetic chords or sutures that can be used to correct degenerative MR with leaflet prolapse usually due to ruptured or torn chordae. The implants are attached to the free end of the MV and anchored to the LV myocardium at the other end. The chords can be delivered via the transapical or transseptal approach. The length of the chords is adjusted to optimize leaflet coaptation. The NeoChord (Minnetonka, MN, USA) and MitraFlex (TransCardiac Therapeutics, Atlanta, GA, USA) systems allow for transapical deployment, with the NeoChord system showing high success rates.[49] The V-Chordal device (Valtech Cardio, Or-Yehuda, Israel) uses the transseptal approach and has the ability to adjust (elongate or shorten) the artificial chordae to achieve optimal coaptation. The concern with all chordal implants is that aggressive therapy may lead to leaflet restriction and residual MR. The presence of material in the intracardiac space may also predispose the patient to thrombus formation.

DISORDERS OF LV DILATION

LV remodeling devices decrease the anterior-posterior dimensions of the LV. Improving LV dimensions reduces the tension on the papillary muscles by bringing them closer to the leaflets and indirectly reduces the septal-lateral annular size improving leaflet coaptation. This approach is used in patients with secondary MR. The iCoapsys system (Myocor, Maple Grove, MN, USA) consists of 2 epicardial pads connected via an intracardiac cord.[50] The device is implanted via an intrapericar-dial catheter through a subxiphoid incision. The Randomized Evaluation of a Surgical Treatment for Off-Pump Repair of the Mitral Valve (RESTOR-MV) trial demonstrated that patients with functional MR requiring revascularization treated with ventric-ular reshaping rather than surgery had improved survival and a significant reduction in major adverse clinical events.[51]

COMBINING PERCUTANEOUS APPROACHES

There are possibilities for combining techniques to improve procedural success at reducing MR. Leaflet plication, space occupiers, and leaflet ablation restore leaflet coaptation but do not address the annular, chordal, or ventricular components of mitral regurgitation. The same holds true with the use of other devices that focus on different anatomic site. They fail to address the other remaining components. Further evaluation of combined approaches is necessary. One device to date, the MitraFlex system, is designed to deploy a clip that captures and approximates the midpoint of the leaflets as well as to implant artifi-cial chordae tendinae. The artificial chordae controls the movement of the valve leaflets and reduces the mitral annular size, helping to restore its saddle-shaped configuration. This device requires a transapical approach and is currently undergoing preclinical testing.

SUMMARY

The MV apparatus is a complex structure with a multitude of faults that cause mitral regurgitation. The pathophysiology of primary and secondary MR is different, as are their options for percuta-neous correction. Transcatheter mitral therapies directed at components of the mitral apparatus (described previously) are available and able to treat different pathophysiologic substrates. The addition of multimodality imaging has further improved treatment of these patients, both by patient selection and guidance during intervention. Overall, percutaneous mitral therapy is evolving and options to treat patients with this complicated disorder are available and intensifying.

REFERENCES

1. Perloff JK, Roberts WC. The mitral apparatus: func-tional anatomy of mitral regurgitation. Circulation 1972;46(2):227–39.
2. Brolin I. The mitral orifice. Acta Radiol Diagn (Stockh) 1967;6(3):273–95.
3. Davis PK, Kinmonth JB. The movements of the annulus of the mitral valve. J Cardiovasc Surg (Torino) 1963;4:427–31.
4. Van Mieghem NM, Piazza N, Anderson RH, et al. Anatomy of the mitral valvular complex and its implications for transcatheter interventions for mitral regurgitation. J Am Coll Cardiol 2010;56(8): 617–26.
5. Delgado V, Tops LF, Schuijf JD, et al. Assessment of mitral valve anatomy and geometry with multislice computed tomography. JACC Cardiovasc Imaging 2009;2(5):556–65.
6. Palazzuoli A, Cademartiri F, Geleijnse ML, et al. Left ventricular remodelling and systolic function measurement with 64 multi-slice computed tomog-raphy versus second harmonic echocardiography in patients with coronary artery disease: a double blind study. Eur J Radiol 2010;73(1):82–8.
7. Ho SY. Anatomy of the mitral valve. Heart 2002; 88(Suppl 4): iv5–10.
8. Levine RA, Triulzi MO, Harrigan P, et al. The relation-ship of mitral annular shape to the diagnosis of mitral valve prolapse. Circulation 1987;75(4):756–67.

9. Korn D, Desanctis RW, Sell S. Massive calcification of the mitral annulus. A clinicopathological study of fourteen cases. N Engl J Med 1962;267:900–9.

10. Montiel MM. Muscular apparatus of the mitral valve in man and its involvement in left-sided cardiac hypertrophy. Am J Cardiol 1970;26(4):341–4.

11. Brock RC. The surgical and pathological anatomy of the mitral valve. Br Heart J 1952;14(4):489–513.

12. Millington-Sanders C, Meir A, Lawrence L, et al. Structure of chordae tendineae in the left ventricle of the human heart. J Anat 1998;192(Pt 4):573–81.

13. Levy MJ, Edwards JE. Anatomy of mitral insufficiency. Prog Cardiovasc Dis 1962;5:119–44.

14. Choure AJ, Garcia MJ, Hesse B, et al. In vivo analysis of the anatomical relationship of coronary sinus to mitral annulus and left circumflex coronary artery using cardiac multidetector computed tomography: implications for percutaneous coronary sinus mitral annuloplasty. J Am Coll Cardiol 2006;48(10):1938–45.

15. Maselli D, Guarracino F, Chiaramonti F, et al. Percutaneous mitral annuloplasty: an anatomic study of human coronary sinus and its relation with mitral valve annulus and coronary arteries. Circulation 2006;114(5):377–80.

16. Tops LF, Van de Veire NR, Schuijf JD, et al. Noninvasive evaluation of coronary sinus anatomy and its relation to the mitral valve annulus: implications for percutaneous mitral annuloplasty. Circulation 2007; 115(11):1426–32.

17. Timek TA, Miller DC. Experimental and clinical assessment of mitral annular area and dynamics: what are we actually measuring? Ann Thorac Surg 2001;72(3):966–74.

18. Carabello BA. The current therapy for mitral regurgitation. J Am Coll Cardiol 2008;52(5):319–26.

19. Trichon BH, Felker GM, Shaw LK, et al. Relation of frequency and severity of mitral regurgitation to survival among patients with left ventricular systolic dysfunction and heart failure. Am J Cardiol 2003; 91(5):538–43.

20. Wu AH, Aaronson KD, Bolling SF, et al. Impact of mitral valve annuloplasty on mortality risk in patients with mitral regurgitation and left ventricular systolic dysfunction. J Am Coll Cardiol 2005; 45(3):381–7.

21. Chiam PT, Ruiz CE. Percutaneous transcatheter mitral valve repair: a classification of the technology. JACC Cardiovasc Interv 2011;4(1):1–13.

22. Foster GP, Dunn AK, Abraham S, et al. Accurate measurement of mitral annular dimensions by echocardiography: importance of correctly aligned imaging planes and anatomic landmarks. J Am Soc Echocardiogr 2009;22(5):458–63.

23. Veronesi F, Corsi C, Sugeng L, et al. Quantification of mitral apparatus dynamics in functional and ischemic mitral regurgitation using real-time 3-dimensional echocardiography. J Am Soc Echocardiogr 2008;21(4):347–54.

24. Grewal J, Mankad S, Freeman WK, et al. Real-time three-dimensional transesophageal echocardiography in the intraoperative assessment of mitral valve disease. J Am Soc Echocardiogr 2009;22(1): 34–41.

25. Sugeng L, Shernan SK, Salgo IS, et al. Live 3-dimensional transesophageal echocardiography initial experience using the fully-sampled matrix array probe. J Am Coll Cardiol 2008;52(6):446–9.

26. De Castro S, Salandin V, Cartoni D, et al. Qualitative and quantitative evaluation of mitral valve morphology by intraoperative volume-rendered three-dimensional echocardiography. J Heart Valve Dis 2002;11(2): 173–80.

27. Ewe SH, Klautz RJ, Schalij MJ, et al. Role of computed tomography imaging for transcatheter valvular repair/insertion. Int J Cardiovasc Imaging 2011. [Epub ahead of print].

28. Feldman T, Wasserman HS, Herrmann HC, et al. Percutaneous mitral valve repair using the edge-to-edge technique: six-month results of the EVEREST Phase I Clinical Trial. J Am Coll Cardiol 2005; 46(11):2134–40.

29. Langerveld J, Valocik G, Plokker HW, et al. Additional value of three-dimensional transesophageal echocardiography for patients with mitral valve stenosis undergoing balloon valvuloplasty. J Am Soc Echocardiogr 2003;16(8):841–9.

30. Shanks M, Delgado V, Ng AC, et al. Mitral valve morphology assessment: three-dimensional transesophageal echocardiography versus computed tomography. Ann Thorac Surg 2010;90(6):1922–9.

31. Hoppe UC, Brandt MC, Degen H, et al. Percutaneous mitral annuloplasty device leaves free access to cardiac veins for resynchronization therapy. Catheter Cardiovasc Interv 2009;74(3):506–11.

32. Schofer J, Siminiak T, Haude M, et al. Percutaneous mitral annuloplasty for functional mitral regurgitation: results of the CARILLON Mitral Annuloplasty Device European Union Study. Circulation 2009;120(4): 326–33.

33. Haude M, Hoppe U, Lipiecki J, et al. Safety and Efficacy Comparison Between Implanted and Non-Implanted Patients in the TITAN Trial using the CARILLON Mitral Contour System to Treat Functional Mitral Regurgitation. TCT. vol. 56. San Francisco, California. J Am Coll Cardiol 2010;B25.

34. Ebner A, Gallo S, Alvarez E, et al. First-in-man percutaneous mitral repair with mitralign. Paper presented at: EuroPCR. Barcelona (Spain), May 2009.

35. Buellesfeld L. Emerging experiences and insights from Mitralign. Paper presented at: TCT. Washington, DC, September 2010.

36. Goel R, Witzel T, Dickens D, et al. The Quantum-Cor device for treating mitral regurgitation: an

animal study. Catheter Cardiovasc Interv 2009; 74(1):43–8.

37. Alfieri O, Maisano F, De Bonis M, et al. The double-orifice technique in mitral valve repair: a simple solution for complex problems. J Thorac Cardiovasc Surg 2001;122(4):674–81.

38. Timek TA, Nielsen SL, Lai DT, et al. Edge-to-edge mitral valve repair without ring annuloplasty for acute ischemic mitral regurgitation. Circulation 2003; 108(Suppl 1):II122–7.

39. Maisano F, Caldarola A, Blasio A, et al. Midterm results of edge-to-edge mitral valve repair without annuloplasty. J Thorac Cardiovasc Surg 2003; 126(6):1987–97.

40. Feldman T, Kar S, Rinaldi M, et al. Percutaneous mitral repair with the MitraClip system: safety and midterm durability in the initial EVEREST (Endovascular Valve Edge-to-Edge REpair Study) cohort. J Am Coll Cardiol 2009;54(8):686–94.

41. Argenziano M, Skipper E, Heimansohn D, et al. Surgical revision after percutaneous mitral repair with the MitraClip device. Ann Thorac Surg 2010; 89(1):72–80 [discussion: p 80].

42. Feldman T, Foster E, Glower DD, et al. Percutaneous repair or surgery for mitral regurgitation. N Engl J Med 2011;364(15):1395–406.

43. Wolfsohn AL, Green MS, Walley VM. Pathology of radiofrequency catheter ablation of the atrioventricular node. Mod Pathol 1994;7(4):494–6.

44. Williams JL, Toyoda Y, Ota T, et al. Feasibility of myxomatous mitral valve repair using direct leaflet and chordal radiofrequency ablation. J Interv Cardiol 2008;21(6):547–54.

45. Davies MJ, Moore BP, Braimbridge MV. The floppy mitral valve. Study of incidence, pathology, and complications in surgical, necropsy, and forensic material. Br Heart J 1978;40(5):468–81.

46. King BD, Clark MA, Baba N, et al. "Myxomatous" mitral valves: collagen dissolution as the primary defect. Circulation 1982;66(2):288–96.

47. Cosgrove DM, Stewart WJ. Mitral valvuloplasty. Curr Probl Cardiol 1989;14(7):359–415.

48. Ye J. Mitra-Spacer: a novel approach to Mitral Regurgitation. Paper presented at: TCT. Washington, DC, September 2010.

49. Seeburger J, Leontjev S, Neumuth M, et al. Transapical beating-heart implantation of neo-chordae to mitral valve leaflets: results of an acute animal study. Eur J Cardiothorac Surg 2011. [Epub ahead of print].

50. Pedersen WR, Block P, Leon M, et al. iCoapsys mitral valve repair system: percutaneous implantation in an animal model. Catheter Cardiovasc Interv 2008;72(1):125–31.

51. Grossi EA, Saunders PC, Woo YJ, et al. Intraoperative effects of the coapsys annuloplasty system in a randomized evaluation (RESTOR-MV) of functional ischemic mitral regurgitation. Ann Thorac Surg 2005;80(5):1706–11.

Percutaneous Techniques for the Treatment of Patients with Functional Mitral Valve Regurgitation

Rodrigo M. Lago, MD, Roberto J. Cubeddu, MD, Igor F. Palacios, MD*

KEYWORDS
- Mitral Valve • Regurgitation • Valvular insufficiency
- Percutaneous device

SCOPE OF THE PROBLEM

Mitral regurgitation (MR) is the most common type of valvular insufficiency. It is estimated that approximately 5 million people in the United States and more than 20 million worldwide suffer from congestive heart failure, often associated with dilated ventricles and coexisting MR. Ischemic cardiomyopathy is the most common cause of heart failure in the United States.[1] This disease is marked by diffuse myocardial damage, left ventricular remodeling, and often functional ischemic MR.[2] Although surgery can be effective in treating MR, it is frequently associated with high operative morbidity, disease recurrence, and increased mortality.[3–5] Currently, potential percutaneous options for the treatment of mitral regurgitation are in different stages of development, either in the early phases of clinical use or being preclinically tested. These techniques are as follows:

- Leaflet coupling with edge-to-edge repair (Evalve MitraClip, Edwards Stitch)
- Coronary sinus reshaping (MONARC device, Carillon device, Miltralife ev3, Cardiac Dimensions, Viacor)
- Annular plication with posterior annulus reshaping (Mitralign, Guided Delivery Systems)
- Left ventricular remodeling (Myocor, Ample PS3 [percutaneous septal sinus shortening]).

This article discusses current options and future directions for the percutaneous treatment of mitral valve regurgitation.

MITRAL VALVE STRUCTURE AND FUNCTION

It is important to understand the anatomic and functional substrate underlying the development of MR. The mitral valve is a complex anatomic structure and its proper function depends on the structural and functional integrity of its individual components (**Fig. 1**). Abnormalities in 1 or more of its components can result in stenosis or regurgitant valvular dysfunction.

The distinction between primary and secondary (functional) MR is important for the potential role of percutaneous device therapies for MR (**Box 1**). In primary organic MR, there is an abnormality of the mitral valve components, whereas in secondary functional MR, the mitral valve itself is

Massachusetts General Hospital, Harvard Medical School, 55 Fruit Street, Boston, MA 02114, USA
* Corresponding author.
E-mail address: ipalacios@partners.org

Intervent Cardiol Clin 1 (2012) 85–99
doi:10.1016/j.iccl.2011.10.001
2211-7458/12/$ – see front matter © 2012 Published by Elsevier Inc.

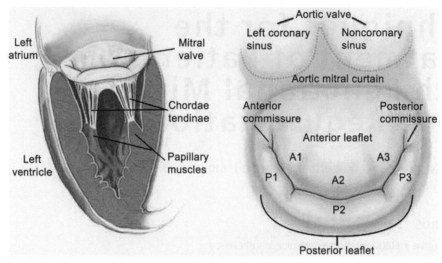

Fig. 1. Anatomy of the mitral valve.

usually unaffected. However, previous damage of the left ventricle (LV) by coronary artery disease or by dilated cardiomyopathy can cause malcoaptation of anatomically normal mitral leaflets in the setting of geometric distortion of the LV, with displacement of papillary muscles and/or annular dilatation with subsequent MR.

Functional MR has been associated with an adverse prognosis among patients with dilated and ischemic cardiomyopathy.[6,7] Although surgical intervention is associated with improved symptoms of heart failure and reverse remodeling of the LV, surgical treatment of functional MR has not been shown to improve survival.[8] Mitral valve repair with reduction annuloplasty rather than replacement is currently favored for the treatment of functional MR.[9,10] Lessons from surgical

experience showed that mitral valve repair can effectively treat many, but not all, patients with functional MR.

Potential factors that can predict the recurrence of MR after mitral repair include the following:

- Annular ring geometry
- Chordae tendineae repositioning
- Concomitant reshaping of the LV during repair
- The need for a complete (D-shaped) annuloplasty ring rather than a partial (C-shaped) ring.[11,12]

Until recently, available treatment options for functional MR were limited to open surgical repair or replacement, an option that is often challenged and associated with high operative morbidity, disease recurrence, and increased mortality.[3–5] The most common form of mitral valve repair involves annuloplasty, the placement of a ring around the mitral annulus to reduce the mitral valve orifice by decreasing the distance between the septal and lateral dimensions of the mitral valve, thereby bringing the leaflet edges closer together. Annuloplasty is used as an adjunctive therapy in most forms of mitral valve repair including functional MR. A less commonly used surgical leaflet repair approach pioneered by Alfieri and colleagues[13] is the edge-to-edge repair that creates a double-orifice mitral valve by suturing the free edges of the mitral leaflets together to form a double orifice. Although the isolated use of this surgical technique has been controversial because of the concomitant use of annuloplasty with most leaflet repairs, follow-up

---

Box 1
Primary and secondary (functional) MR

Primary organic MR
- Abnormality of the mitral valve components

Secondary functional MR
- Mitral valve usually unaffected
- Previous damage of the LV (by coronary artery disease or by dilated cardiomyopathy) can cause malcoaptation of anatomically normal mitral leaflets in the setting of geometric distortion of the LV, with displacement of papillary muscles and/or annular dilatation with subsequent MR

for as long as 12 years in patients who have undergone isolated surgical edge-to-edge repair without annuloplasty has shown durable clinical outcome with this surgical technique.[13,14] In the past decade, potential percutaneous catheter-based treatment strategies for valvular heart disease have emerged as an attractive option. Percutaneous therapies for MR try to emulate surgical approaches that have been in use for many years.

PERCUTANEOUS TREATMENT OF MITRAL VALVE REGURGITATION

In general, there are 4 groups of strategies for transcatheter treatment of MR:

1. Leaflet coupling with edge-to-edge repair to simulate the Alfieri stitch procedure[15–17]
2. Coronary sinus reshaping devices (indirect annuloplasty)
3. Annular plication with posterior annulus reshaping (direct annuloplasty)
4. Left ventricular remodeling devices (**Table 1**).

PERCUTANEOUS EDGE-TO-EDGE REPAIR

The Alfieri surgical technique to treat degenerative and functional MR was introduced in the early 1990s by Alfieri and colleagues.[13] Although initially poorly accepted, the Alfieri stitch or edge-to-edge technique gained popularity.[18] The technique consisted of suturing the free edges of the middle anterior (A2) and posterior (P2) mitral leaflets and creating a double-orifice inlet valve. The technique was intended to improve leaflet coaptation and therefore decrease MR. Long-term results from this technique were reported for both degenerative and functional MR with 5-year freedom from recurrent MR more than 2+ and reoperation rates as

high as 90%.[19] The development of transcatheter mitral valve edge-to-edge repair techniques was based on the surgical technique. Two mitral valve percutaneous techniques and devices have been developed to emulate the double-orifice strategy using a catheter-based approach: the Evalve MitraClip (Evalve Inc., Menlo Park, CA, USA) and the MOBIUS system (Edwards Lifesciences Corp., Irvine, CA, USA).

The Evalve MitraClip

The Evalve MitraClip (**Fig. 2**) is a device that uses a guide catheter that is placed using transseptal puncture, a delivery catheter, and an implantable 4-mm-wide cobalt-chromium implant clip with 2 arms covered with polyester fabric (see **Fig. 2**). The device uses a triaxial catheter system to deliver its clip fixation device and create a double-orifice mitral valve.

After the initial encouraging results in animal models, this transcatheter technique was first used in humans in 2003. During 2-year follow-up after MitraClip implantation, a 56-year-old woman with heart failure and severe 4+ MR remained asymptomatic with less than 2+ MR.[20,21]

The safety and feasibility of the MitraClip system were tested in the EVEREST (Endovascular Valve Edge-to-Edge Repair Study) phase I and phase II studies.[22] Results from the 107 patients (55 from EVEREST I; 52 from EVEREST II) with either degenerative (79%) or functional (21%) MR were encouraging. On an intent-to-treat basis, implant success occurred in 90% of patients, in whom acute success (MR grade ≤2+) was reported in 84% of the cases. Among these patients, improvement in New York Heart Association (NYHA) functional class was reported in 73% at 1-year

Table 1
Current status of percutaneous mitral valve repair procedures

Approach	Device	Manufacturer
Edge-to-edge leaflet repair	MitraClip MOBIUS	Evalve Edwards Lifesciences
Indirect annuloplasty	Carillon PTMA MitraLife MONARC	Cardiac Dimensions Viacor ev3 Edwards Lifesciences
Direct annuloplasty	Mitralign Accucinch QuantumCor	Mitralign Guided Delivery Systems QuantumCor
Ventricular remodeling	iCoapsys	Myocor
Atrial/coronary sinus remodeling	PS3 PMVR	Ample Medical St Jude Medical

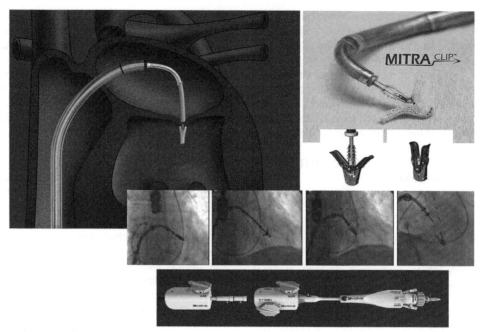

Fig. 2. Evalve MitraClip.

follow-up. Partial clip detachment occurred in 9% of the initial cohort and was the most important mechanical problem with the procedure. This complication was often detected at the protocol-mandated 30-day echocardiogram. These partial detachments were generally not associated with symptoms, and most were treated either with surgery or second clip placement.

Midterm durability of the MitraClip in the EVEREST study has recently been reported and showed low rates of morbidity and mortality and acute MR reduction to less than or equal to 2+ in most patients.[23] The initial 107 patients were analyzed. Nine percent had a major adverse event, including 1 death not related to the procedure. There were no clip embolizations. Partial clip detachment occurred in 9% of patients. Overall, 74% of the patients achieved acute procedural success, and 64% were discharged with MR of less than or equal to 1+. During the 3.2 years after MitraClip implantations, 30% of the patients underwent mitral valve surgery. When surgical mitral valve repair was planned, 84% (21 of 25 patients) were successful. Thus, surgical options were preserved. A total of 66% of the successfully treated patients were free from death, mitral valve surgery, or MR greater than or equal to 2+ at 12 months, which was the primary efficacy end point of the study. Freedom from death was 95.9%, 94.0%, and 90.1%, and freedom from surgery was 88.5%, 83.2%, and 76.3% at 1, 2, and 3 years, respectively. Similar acute results and durability were

observed among the 23 patients with functional MR enrolled in the study.

A recently reported hemodynamic substudy of EVEREST showed that successful mitral valve repair with the MitraClip system resulted in an immediate and significant improvement in the following:

- Forward stroke volume
- Cardiac output
- Left ventricular loading conditions.

There was no evidence of a low cardiac output state following MitraClip treatment of MR, a complication occasionally observed after surgical mitral valve repair for severe MR.[24]

The EVEREST II trial, a prospective, randomized, phase II, multicenter study between the United States and Canada comparing MitraClip with either surgical valve repair or replacement in 279 patients randomized in a 2-to-1 fashion. Twelve-month follow-up showed that, despite being driven by a higher incidence of blood transfusions in the surgical group, safety end points were reached in about 50% of surgery patients and 15% of MitraClip patients, showing superiority of safety for the percutaneous approach by intention to treat. The 1-year efficacy end point of the combined incidence of death, mitral valve surgery, or reoperation for mitral valve dysfunction was more frequent in the surgery patients than in the MitraClip patients, meeting the noninferiority hypothesis for efficacy. Similar reductions in left ventricular volumes and dimensions, and improvements in NYHA functional class, were achieved in both groups after 1 year.

Careful evaluation and patient selection is critical for the success of the procedure. Patients with degenerative or functional MR are candidates for the procedure. Patient selection criteria are shown in **Box 2**.

Technically, the procedure is performed with general anesthesia, using fluoroscopy and transesophageal echocardiography (TEE). Transseptal access is used to place a guide catheter into the left atrium. The Evalve MitraClip guide catheter is 24 Fr proximally and tapers to 22 Fr distally at the level of the atrial septum. It is inserted from the femoral vein and advanced above the mitral valve following a transseptal puncture. The steering knob at the end of the guide allows flexion and lateral movement of the distal tip so that the clip is positioned orthogonally over the 3 planes of the mitral valve and the origin of the regurgitant jet. The delivery catheter passes coaxially through the guide, and has the MitraClip attached to its distal end. The clip arms are opened and closed by a knob on the delivery catheter handle. The opened span of the clip is approximately 2 cm and the width is 4 mm. Through the guide catheter, the delivery system is maneuvered to center the clip over the mitral orifice, and the clip is partially opened and passed across the leaflets into the LV. The open clip is then pulled back to grasp the mitral leaflets and the clip is closed. The degree of MR is assessed by TEE. If necessary, the clip is reopened, the mitral leaflets released, and the clip repositioned. If needed, a second clip is placed. Once optimal reduction of MR is achieved, the clip is released from the delivery system and both the delivery system and guide catheter are withdrawn. Repeat hemodynamic, angiographic, and echocardiographic assessments are routinely performed. Heparin is routinely used during the procedure and administered to achieve an activated clotting time of 250 seconds or more. Aspirin 325 mg and clopidogrel 75 mg daily are ordinarily recommended following the procedure for 6 months and 30 days respectively. Clip failure is well tolerated and does not preclude surgical mitral valve repair or replacement.

The MOBIUS Leaflet Repair System

The MOBIUS leaflet repair system (Edwards Lifesciences Inc., Irvine, CA, USA), also called Milano Stitch, (**Fig. 3**) was introduced by Buchbinder and colleagues as a similar catheter-based edge-to-edge technique. In contrast with the Evalve MitraClip, this strategy uses a small guiding catheter to stitch the free edges of the anterior and the posterior mitral leaflets, thus creating a double-orifice inlet valve. An innovative suction catheter is used to bring the leaflets together and facilitate stitch placement under fluoroscopic and echocardiographic guidance.[25]

After the successful animal model experience, the first in-human case was performed in Milan, Italy, in a 67-year-old woman with NYHA functional class III and severe (grade 4+) MR secondary to a prolapsed posterior leaflet. Subsequently, the percutaneous Alfieri-like stitch was tested in a feasibility trial of 15 patients with either degenerative or functional MR. In this phase I study, acute procedure success occurred in 9 of 15 patients. Of these, 3 patients required a single stitch, 5 required 2 stitches, and 1 patient required 3 stitches. At 30-day follow-up, only 66% of the patients (6 of 9) had a successful stitch in place with at least 1 grade improvement in MR reduction. The patients with acute failure (6 of 15) all underwent subsequent successful surgical repair. However, the study's intermediate result has prompted the investigators to abandon further evaluation for this indication.

PERCUTANEOUS ANNULOPLASTY

Annuloplasty is the mainstay of surgery in patients with functional MR. Annular dilation caused by dilation of the LV and geometric distortion of the mitral apparatus is the mechanism of MR in this group of patients. Surgical mitral annuloplasty typically involves a complete ring to reshape the mitral annulus. Partial annuloplasty is thought to be ineffective. Percutaneous annuloplasty approaches are either direct or indirect (**Box 3**).

Indirect approaches use the coronary sinus as a route to deliver a device to partially wrap the mitral annulus parallel to the posterior mitral valve

---

Box 2
Patient selection criteria for Evalve MitraClip implantation

- Coaptation length of at least 2 mm
- With a flail mitral leaflet, a flail gap less than or equal to 10 mm or a flail width on short-axis estimation less than 15 mm
- MR jet must arise from the central two-thirds of the line of coaptation as seen on short-axis color Doppler examination
- Baseline mitral valve area should be greater than 4 cm² to avoid the creation of mitral stenosis

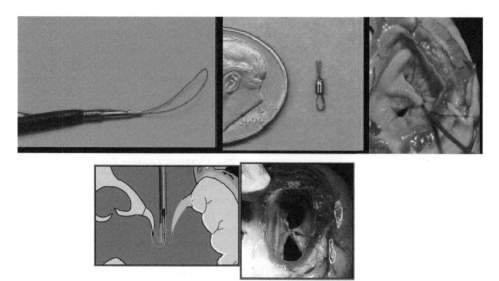

Fig. 3. Milano Stitch/MOBIUS device.

leaflet and create tension that is transmitted to the mitral annulus. The rationale is that any conformation change of the coronary sinus may be used advantageously to reduce the septal-lateral annular dimensions and improve MR severity. Indirect annuloplasty approaches include the Cardiac Dimensions Carillon system (Cardiac Dimensions, Kirkland, WA, USA), the Edwards MONARC system (Edwards Lifesciences, Irvine, CA, USA), the MitraLife/ev3 device, and the Viacor PTMA (percutaneous transvenous mitral annuloplasty) system (Viacor, Wilmington, MA, USA).

Direct annuloplasty approaches involve direct implantation of a device into the mitral annulus, which more closely mimics surgical annuloplasty.

Direct annuloplasty devices include the Mitralign system (Mitralign, Tewksbury, MA, USA) and the Guided Delivery Systems device (Guided Delivery Systems, Santa Clara, CA, USA).

Indirect Annuloplasty Techniques

Cardiac dimensions carillon device

The Cardiac Dimensions Carillon device (Cardiac Dimensions, Kirkland, WA, USA) (**Fig. 4**) system combines an implantable device and delivery system. The device consists of 2 anchors connected by a nitinol bridge.

Via jugular access under fluoroscopic guidance, a 9-Fr guide catheter is delivered into the distal coronary sinus. A distal anchor is placed in the great cardiac vein and a proximal anchor is placed near the ostium of the coronary sinus. Once the distal anchor is deployed into the great cardiac vein, tension is applied to the system resulting in immediate decrease in the diameter of the mitral annulus, by moving the posterior leaflet more anteriorly. Then, the proximal anchor is released. Simultaneous TEE allows for direct visualization of MR improvement.

The Carillon Mitral Contour System is simple, quick, and easy to use. It is adjustable and can apply varying degrees of tension to a system. It is compatible, because it fits contours of various anatomies, allowing for optimal and safe delivery to occur. A major advantage of this device is that it is retrievable if positioning is not optimal. Its intuitive delivery system comes in sizes of 60 mm in length with a distal anchor height of 7 to 14 mm and proximal anchor height of 12 to 20 mm (1.5–2.0 ratios). The issue with the first generation of the device, in which there was a difficulty in

---

Box 3
Percutaneous annuloplasty approaches

Indirect annuloplasty approaches

Cardiac Dimensions Carillon system (Cardiac Dimensions, Kirkland, WA, USA)

Edwards MONARC system (Edwards Lifesciences, Irvine, CA, USA)

MitraLife/ev3 device

Viacor PTMA (percutaneous transvenous mitral annuloplasty) system (Viacor, Wilmington, MA, USA)

Direct annuloplasty devices

Mitralign system (Mitralign, Tewksbury, MA, USA)

Guided Delivery Systems device (Guided Delivery Systems, Santa Clara, CA, USA)

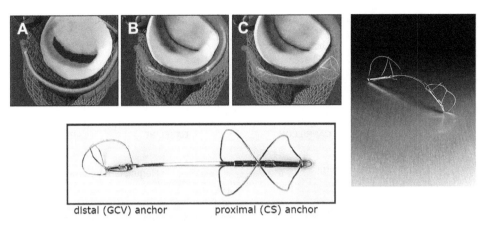

distal (GCV) anchor   proximal (CS) anchor

Fig. 4. The Carillon system consists of a nitinol bridge connecting a distal anchor that is placed at the greater cardiac vein and a proximal anchor placed in the proximal coronary sinus. (*A*) Delivery system in the CS; (*B*) Deployment of the Carillon system into the CS around the mitral valve annulus; (*C*) Carilon system deployed in position into the CS. CS, coronary sinus; GCV, great cardiac vein.

anchoring, was corrected with improvements in engineering (Carillon XE).

Initial experiments in animals showed that placement of the Carillon system in 6 dogs with dilated cardiomyopathy resulted in both a mean decrease in mitral annulus diameter from 2.7 ($\pm$ 0.2) cm to 2.3 ($\pm$0.1) cm ($P<.05$), and a mean decrease in MR/left atrial area ratio from 16 ($\pm$4) to 4 ($\pm$1) ($P = .052$).[26] The first in-human implantation of the Carillon device was performed by Dr Schofer in Hamburg, Germany.

Recently, the AMADEUS (Carillon Mitral Annuloplasty Device European Union Study) trial, a prospective, single-arm, multicenter safety and efficacy trial of the Carillon system, was reported. The primary end point of the study was safety of deployment and implantation of the device in the coronary sinus and the great cardiac vein. The secondary end point included long-term safety and effect of the device on hemodynamic parameters and subject function.

The study enrolled 48 patients with follow-up at intervals of 1, 3, and 6 months. Candidate patients with CHF, MR ($\geq$2+), and decreased left ventricular systolic function (ejection fraction <40%) for the trial underwent a standardized 6-minute walking test, a TEE, a treadmill test, and a multislice computed tomography scan to determine the anatomic relationship between the coronary sinus, the mitral annulus ring, and the left circumflex coronary artery. Angiographic examination of the coronary sinus and the coronary arteries were acquired before device implantation. The study initially enrolled 4 patients between July 2005 and March 2006, and showed successful permanent device implantation in only 1 patient. This patient had successful reductions in MR

severity and improvement in functional status that persisted at 6 months' follow-up. In the remaining 3 patients, the device moved because the distal anchor was unable to consistently maintain its shape during device tensioning before final deployment. Nevertheless, the devices were recaptured and removed safely. Successful implantation occurred in 70% of the patients, and resulted in improved functional class and MR severity of at least 1+ in 80% of the cases. Those who benefited most had evidence of congestive heart failure and greater than or equal to 2+ centric MR secondary to mitral annulus dilatation. Acute MR reduction (grade 3.0 $\pm$ 0.6 to 2.0 $\pm$ 0.8, $P<.0001$) and permanent implantation were achieved in 30 of 43 patients in whom an attempt was made. Additional measurements in 20 patients with implants showed reductions in the vena contracta (0.69 $\pm$ 0.29–0.46 $\pm$ 0.26 cm, $P<.0001$), effective regurgitant orifice area (0.33 $\pm$ 0.17–0.19 $\pm$ 0.08 cm^2, $P<.0001$), regurgitant volume (40 $\pm$ 20–24 $\pm$ 11 mL, $P = .0005$), and jet area/left atrial area (45% $\pm$ 13%–32% $\pm$ 12%, $P<.0001$) (**Fig. 5**). The coronary arteries were crossed in 36 patients (84%) (see **Fig. 5**).

One major limitation of this device is the potential obstruction of left circumflex coronary artery flow during device deployment. In 84% of the patients, the device crossed the left circumflex coronary artery, in which compromise of blood flow occurred in 14%, and in whom the device was immediately retrieved. Overall, the AMADEUS study achieved its safety end point with an acceptable adverse event profile. MR was reduced by 27% out to 6 months and the patients had significant improvements in functional parameters out to 6 months.[27]

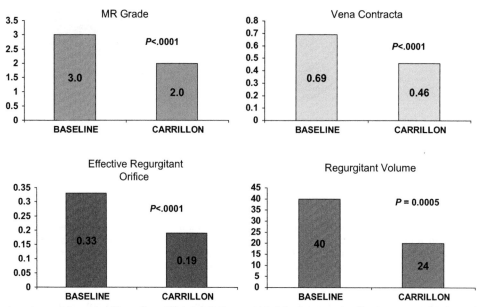

Fig. 5. Amadeus trial results. (*Data from* Siminiak T, Hoppe UC, Schofer J, et al. Effectiveness and safety of percutaneous coronary sinus-based mitral valve repair in patients with dilated cardiomyopathy (from the AMADEUS trial). Am J Cardiol 2009;104(4):565–70.)

Edwards MONARC system

The Edwards MONARC system (Edwards Lifesciences, Irvine, CA, USA) is percutaneously implanted in the coronary sinus after cannulation with a guide catheter. The device is designed to improve MR severity over an estimated period of 3 to 6 weeks, remodeling the mitral annulus by implanting a bioabsorbable springlike bridge that is connected between 2 self-expanding proximal and distal nitinol stents (**Fig. 6**).

The procedure is performed under local anesthesia via a 12-Fr right transjugular approach.

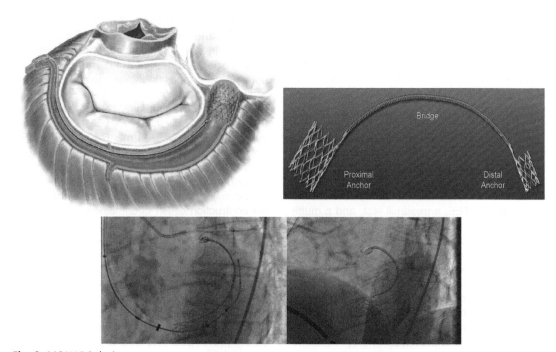

Fig. 6. MONARC device.

The stent anchors provide force that brings the proximal coronary sinus and distal great cardiac vein together while the interconnecting bridge tenses and foreshortens with time. The conformational changes invoked over the posterior annular segment presumably shorten the septal-lateral dimensions to reduce MR severity.

The first human experience with the MONARC system was reported by Webb and colleagues[28] in 2006 and included 5 patients with chronic severe ischemic MR. Implantation was successful in 4 of the 5 patients, and resulted in a mean decrease in MR grade from 3+ to 1+. Loss of efficacy was later seen in 3 of the patients, caused by asymptomatic separation and fracture of the bridging segment.

Following device modification and reinforcement of the bridging segment, the EVOLUTION (Clinical Evaluation of the Edwards Lifesciences Percutaneous Mitral Annuloplasty System for the Treatment of Mitral Regurgitation) phase I study was conducted. In this study, successful implantation was achieved in 59 of the 72 patients (82%) with functional MR and heart failure. Freedom from death, MI, and cardiac tamponade at 30 days was 91%. Left circumflex coronary artery compression occurred in 30% of patients. Major adverse events at 18-months included 1 death, 3 myocardial infarctions, 2 coronary sinus perforations, 1 anchor displacement, and 4 anchor separations. This study showed that implantation of the MONARC system was feasible, and, although efficacy data are encouraging, coronary compression and anchor separations remain important concerns and limitations. The effect of the Edwards MONARC device cannot be assessed at the time of placement, therefore there is no indication regarding the efficacy outcome until the spring has shortened several weeks later. The EVOLUTION II trial study of the MONARC device has been stopped by the sponsor because of slow enrollment.

Viacor PTMA system

The Viacor PTMA system (**Fig. 7**) consists of a polytetrafluoroethylene catheter in which rods of different stiffness are introduced into the distal part of the coronary sinus via subclavian or jugular venous puncture. A trilumen plastic cannula is delivered into the coronary sinus and nitinol rods are passed through the lumens of the catheter to apply pressure to the posterior annulus in the central part of the posterior mitral valve leaflet (P2) and compress the septolateral dimension. Following the identification of the optimal amount of compression of the posterior annulus to result in a reduction in MR, permanent implantation is performed. The device can be retrieved in cases of absence of reduction in MR or left coronary circumflex cinching.[29–31] Preliminary studies in sheep models were highly encouraging and resulted in decreased MR severity from between +3 and +4 to between +0 and +1 ($P<.03$), and associated with significant reductions in septal-lateral mitral annular dimensions (from 30 ± 2.1 mm to 24 ± 1.7 mm; $P<.03$).[32] The first in-human feasibility and safety study was reported in 2007 and included 4 patients with ischemic MR and NYHA class II or III, MR greater than or equal to 2+, type I and/or IIIB Carpentier MR functional class requiring surgical mitral annuloplasty, and showed continued reduction of the mitral orifice for as long as 1 year after initial implantation. In this study, the device was temporarily implanted, adjusted, and subsequently removed. The investigators report substantial reductions in regurgitant volumes (45.5 ± 24.4 to 13.3 ± 7.3 mL) caused by the mechanically induced anterior-posterior diameter

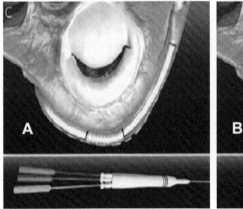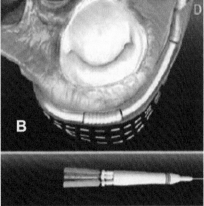

Fig. 7. The Viacor PTMA system consists of a catheter with nitinol rods of different stiffness introduced into the distal part of the coronary sinus (*A*) to apply pressure at the posterior mitral valve annulus (*B*).

reduction (40.75 ± 4.3 to 35.2 ± 1.6 mm) in 3 patients. In 1 patient, the device could not be deployed because of extreme angulated anatomy.[30] Recently, the Canadian and European phase I PTOLEMY (Percutaneous Transvenous Mitral Annuloplasty) trial has been reported. This study included 27 patients with NYHA functional class II or III, and moderate to severe functional MR.[33] Successful implantation was performed in 19 of the 27 patients. The remainder were excluded because of unsuitable coronary sinus anatomy. Of those who underwent successful implantation, 13 had a reduction in MR severity and, in 6, the device was ineffective. Device removal was required in 4 patients because of fracture, device migration, or diminished efficacy. Long-term success in MR reduction was seen in only 18.5% of the patients. An attractive feature of this device is the ability to regain venous access at a later date to remove rods if the reduction of MR is diminished. In that case, stiffer rods may be used to replace the initial implanted rods. The phase II PTOLEMY trial has been presented and showed 2.8% 30-day cardiac event rates and greater than 90% procedural success. However, the company has stopped further development and manufacturing of the device.

Despite the effectiveness and ease of use of the coronary sinus devices approach, they all have limitations. Metal fatigue and the risk of device fracture caused by mechanical stress in the coronary sinus created by torsional forces on these devices is an important issue. Reengineering of all of these devices has improved outcomes. A second limitation common to this class of device is the potential for compression of the left circumflex coronary artery. Cardiac computed tomography to assess the relationship of the coronary sinus and the coronary arteries before device implantation is an important step in the evaluation of these patients before annular device implantation.

MitraLife device

The MitraLife device (ev3/Edwards Lifesciences, Irvine, CA, USA) is one of the first annuloplasty devices tested in humans. It consists of a percutaneous delivery system that is preloaded with the MitraLife device and is permanently implanted in the coronary sinus via the internal jugular approach. The device is designed to reduce mitral annular size and restore valve leaflet closure. Durability and feasibility results in canine animal models have thus far been promising, and have been associated with significant reduction in MR. To date, only a handful of human temporary placements have occurred outside the Unites States.

Initial reports of the MitraLife device have been presented of 7 patients (5 men and 2 women), aged 22 to 66 years, with functional MR. All patients had severe MR and NYHC III and IV, and the mean ejection fraction was 27%. Significant reductions in mitral annulus and MR were described; however, a clinical trial is pending.

Direct Annuloplasty Techniques

Mitralign system

The Mitralign system (Mitralign, Tewksbury, MA, USA) involves placement of the guide catheter under the middle scallop of the posterior mitral leaflet. The device consists of a deflectable catheter that is manipulated and advanced in a retrograde fashion across the aortic valve through a 14-Fr femoral sheath into the subvalvular mitral valve space. A steerable catheter with a deflectable 2-arm (bident) catheter end is delivered via a 12.5-Fr guide catheter between the papillary muscles facing the posterior mitral annulus. Once properly aligned, anchor pledgets are delivered from the LV to the left atrium across the circumferential mitral valve annulus and pulled together with a guidewire to decrease the annulus septal-lateral dimension. The feasibility and durability of this technique has been confirmed in early animal studies in which significant reductions in MR were shown.[34] Currently, the technique is being tested in a safety and feasibility phase I clinical study; however, preliminary results have yet to be released and clinical outcome data are expected in the future.

Accucinch device

The Accucinch device (Guided Delivery Systems, Santa Clara, CA, USA) is another promising strategy. A small adjustable ring of anchors interlinked with a cable is implanted percutaneously into the muscle below the mitral valve. The cinching effect improves the ability of the mitral valve to close properly and reduces the mitral regurgitation. After access to the annulus, a series of as many as 12 nitinol anchors are placed in the mitral annulus. These anchors are connected with a cord that is tensioned to draw the anchors together. This device has been implanted surgically, and first-in-human experience has shown the technical feasibility of percutaneous use. The Accucinch system has been successfully tested during open heart surgery in 2 patients with 2+ MR and coronary arterial disease undergoing routine coronary artery bypass grafting. The surgically implanted device resulted in sustained and successful reductions in MR severity at 6-month and 12-month follow-up. The first in-human percutaneous implantation of the Accucinch system for mitral valve repair was reported in 2009. The procedure was performed by Dr Schofer in Hamburg, Germany, and the Accucinch system significantly reduced the patient's mitral regurgitation.

Although arterial access as the delivery route adds morbidity to the procedure compared with the simplicity and ease of use of the transvenous coronary sinus approach, direct annuloplasty has the advantage of avoiding coronary compression, and the potential for greater efficacy in reduction of MR through the direct approach is highly attractive. Direct annuloplasty technologies are in early development, and more human experience is expected.

QuantumCor system

The QuantumCor system (QuantumCor Inc., Lake Forest, CA, USA) (**Fig. 8**) represents a unique and different concept that has yet to be tested in humans. This technology is based on thermal remodeling of collagen (TRC), which uses the high collagen content of the mitral valve annulus in which high-frequency energy is delivered through an electrode to denature collagen fibers, causing them to shrink and consequently remodeling the annulus. The end-loop catheter electrode system device is positioned on the dilated valve annulus where a precise subablative radiofrequency energy protocol is delivered. This protocol releases the hydrogen bonds in the collagen fibers of the mitral annulus, causing them to shrink. The posterior annulus is treated in 4 quadrants from trigone to trigone, achieving segmental shrinkage in each quadrant. Segmental shrinkage in all 4 quadrants results in a remodeling of the valve annulus, a reduction of the anteroposterior dimension of the valve, and improved coaptation of the valve leaflets. When the procedure is complete, the catheter device is removed and no hardware is left in the heart or vascular system. The technique has been tested in acute and chronic sheep models in which up to 20% reductions in septal-lateral annular dimensions have been reported.[35] Histopathologic examination has shown no evidence of undesirable injury to related structures.

REMODELING OF THE LEFT VENTRICULAR/LEFT ATRIAL MITRAL VALVULAR COMPLEX

This group of transcatheter devices is currently being developed to improve the paravalvular geometric distortion that is encountered in patients with functional MR.

PS3

The PS3 system (Ample Medical, Inc.) (**Fig. 9**) is a transcatheter atrial/mitral annulus remodeling device that integrates several concepts and consists of an atrial septal occluder, an interconnecting cinching wire, and a permanent small coronary sinus T-bar element that is positioned behind P2. The interatrial occluder serves as a pivotal anchor and allows cinching to occur from the posterior annulus to the superior medial interatrial septum. The concept was based on previous animal studies that showed increase in posterior wall to interatrial septum dimensions in functional MR. The initial experience with the PS3 device was first reported in 23 sheep with dilated cardiomyopathy and functional MR. Immediate and midterm results at 30 days revealed important reductions in septal to lateral dimensions and MR severity.[36] Coronary arterial impingement was not observed, and the great cardiac vein was patent in all animals during follow-up histopathologic examination. Significant hemodynamic improvements and a reduction in brain natriuretic peptide levels were observed. The feasibility and safety of this technique was first confirmed in 2 patients undergoing temporary implantation of the PS3 system before mitral valve repair surgery.[37] In the first patient, the PS3 resulted in a relative change of 29% in septal-lateral dimension and was associated with a 1+ decrease in MR severity. The MR severity in the

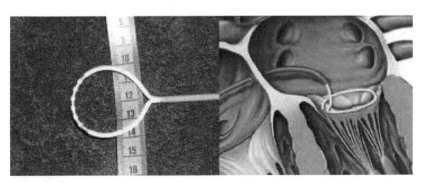

Fig. 8. QuantumCor device.

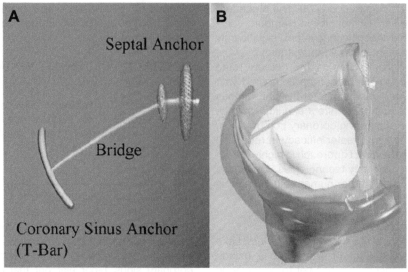

Fig. 9. (*A*) The PS3 device consists of a septal anchor, a bridge, and a coronary sinus anchor. (*B*) PS3 device in place.

second patient decreased from +3 to +1 following a 31% relative change in septal-lateral dimension. No procedural complications were reported. The ongoing CAFÉ trial is a phase I safety and feasibility study of long-term PS3 implantation in humans with heart failure and severe functional MR.

The iCoapsys Left Ventricular Reshaping Device

The iCoapsys (Myocor Inc., Maple Grove, MN, USA) left ventricular reshaping device was, until recently, a promising alternative percutaneous strategy developed to treat functional MR

(**Fig. 10**). Although no longer in use, the strategy represents an important concept. The iCoapsys transventricular system consists of an anterior and posterior epicardial pad tethered together by a subvalvular transventricular chord that travels through the LV and between the papillary muscles. After its implantation via subxyphoid pericardial approach, the chord length can be reduced and adjusted to establish optimal septal-lateral LV and annular dimensions. Conformational changes are intended to reorient the papillary muscles and reduce LV geometric distortion, resulting in a decrease in regurgitant orifice and MR severity. Promising results were reported from

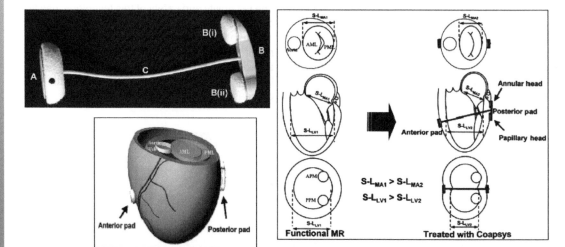

Fig. 10. The iCoapsys transventricular device and its mechanical reconfiguration of the left ventricle to treat functional mitral regurgitation. AML, anterior mitral valve leaflet, APL, anterior papillary muscle, PML, posterior mitral valve leaflet; PPM, posterior papillary muscle, S-L$_{LV}$, septal-lateral left ventricle; S-L$_{MA}$, septal-lateral mitral annulus, (before [1] and after [2] device implantation).

the early animal experience.[38] Unfortunately, the VIVID (Valvular and Ventricular Improvement Via iCoapsys Delivery) feasibility study in humans was prematurely discontinued because of technical difficulties during device implantation and suboptimal patient applicability.

PERIVALVULAR PROSTHETIC MITRAL REGURGITATION

Percutaneous repair of perivalvular prosthetic mitral regurgitation has evolved to become another important and attractive alternative to surgical correction. Paravalvular mitral regurgitation is a serious complication seen in up to 7% of patients following prosthetic heart valve surgery.[39,40] In this group of patients, redo-operations are commonly associated with increased procedural mortality.[41] More recently, percutaneous endovascular devices have been evaluated with promising results.[42–44] The Amplatzer Vascular Plug, the Septal Occluder, and Duct Occluder (AGA Medical Inc., Golden Valley, MN, USA) are used to seal the paravalvular regurgitation. The Amplatzer Duct Occluder is the most commonly used device. Implantation of 2 or more devices may be

necessary. In our experience, simultaneous three-dimensional (3D) TEE imaging should be encouraged for all cases, because it provides optimal information during device implantation (**Fig. 11**).[45]

SUMMARY AND FUTURE DIRECTIONS

Percutaneous approaches to MR remain largely investigational. However, in the last decade, novel percutaneous strategies have opened new options in the treatment of valvular heart disease. Animal and early human studies indicate that many of these techniques are safe and feasible. Several important clinical studies are currently underway to determine the benefits of transcatheter mitral valve repair therapy. Given the complexity of the mitral valve apparatus and its subvalvular structure, a single device to treat all forms of mitral regurgitation is unlikely to be effective in every patient. However, the encouraging results of the MitraClip suggests that this technique may eventually play an important role in the treatment of organic MR. In contrast, the role for isolated coronary sinus devices remains uncertain. The role of transcatheter left ventricular remodeling devices to treat functional MR is at the beginning of its

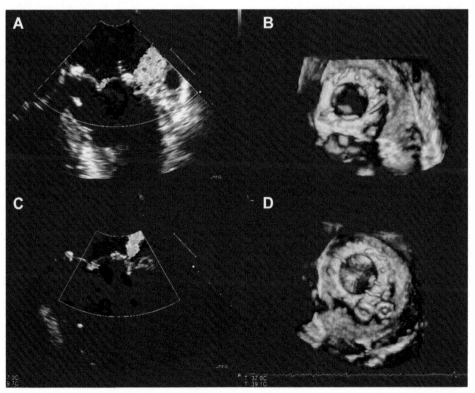

Fig. 11. Doppler and 3D echocardiographic imaging of a mitral paravalvular leak before (*A, B*) and after (*C, D*) successful transcatheter closure using 2 Amplatzer Occluder PDA devices.

development. Transcatheter chordal procedures are being developed, including chordal cutting and chordal implantatation.[46,47] Transcatheter valve implantation in the mitral position might offer a desirable alternative in selected patients and has been accomplished in a compassionate fashion on rare occasions in patients who are not candidates for surgical valve repair or replacement.

REFERENCES

1. Gheorghiade M, Sopko G, De Luca L, et al. Navigating the crossroads of coronary artery disease and heart failure. Circulation 2006;114:1202–13.
2. Sutton MG, Sharpe N. Left ventricular remodeling after myocardial infarction: pathophysiology and therapy. Circulation 2000;101:2981–8.
3. McGee EC, Gillinov AM, Blackstone EH, et al. Recurrent mitral regurgitation after annuloplasty for functional ischemic mitral regurgitation. J Thorac Cardiovasc Surg 2004;128(6):916–24.
4. Gillinov AM, Wierup PN, Blackstone EH, et al. Is repair preferable to replacement for ischemic mitral regurgitation? J Thorac Cardiovasc Surg 2001; 122(6):1125–41.
5. Grossi EA, Goldberg JD, LaPietra A, et al. Ischemic mitral valve reconstruction and replacement: comparison of long-term survival and complications. J Thorac Cardiovasc Surg 2001;122(6):1107–24.
6. Koelling TM, Aaronson KD, Cody RJ, et al. Prognostic significance of mitral regurgitation and tricuspid regurgitation in patients with left ventricular systolic dysfunction. Am Heart J 2002;144:524–9.
7. Bursi F, Enriquez-Sarano M, Nkomo VT, et al. Heart failure and death after myocardial infarction in the community: the emerging role of mitral regurgitation. Circulation 2005;111:295–301.
8. Wu AH, Aaronson KD, Bolling SF, et al. Impact of mitral valve annuloplasty on mortality risk in patients with mitral regurgitation and left ventricular systolic dysfunction. J Am Coll Cardiol 2005; 45:381–7.
9. Bolling SF, Pagani FD, Deeb GM, et al. Intermediate-term outcome of mitral reconstruction in cardiomyopathy. J Thorac Cardiovasc Surg 1998;115:381–8.
10. Bax JJ, Braun J, Somer ST, et al. Restrictive annuloplasty and coronary revascularization in ischemic mitral regurgitation results in reverse left ventricular remodeling. Circulation 2004;110(Suppl):II-103–8.
11. Hueb AC, Jatene FB, Moreira LFP, et al. Ventricular remodeling and mitral valve modifications in dilated cardiomyopathy: new insights from anatomic study. J Thorac Cardiovasc Surg 2002;124:1216–24.
12. Kaji S, Nasu M, Yamamuro A, et al. Annular geometry in patients with chronic ischemic mitral regurgitation: three-dimensional magnetic resonance imaging study. Circulation 2005;112(Suppl):I-409–14.
13. Alfieri O, Maisano F, De Bonis M, et al. The double-orifice technique in mitral valve repair: a simple solution for complex problems. J Thorac Cardiovasc Surg 2001;122(4):674–81.
14. Maisano F, Viganò G, Blasio A, et al. Surgical isolated edge-to-edge mitral valve repair without annuloplasty: clinical proof of the principle for an endovascular approach. EuroIntervention 2006;2: 181–6.
15. Alfieri O, Maisano F, DeBonis M, et al. The edge-to-edge technique in mitral valve repair: a simple solution for complex problems. J Thorac Cardiovasc Surg 2001;122:674–81.
16. Maisano F, Torracca L, Oppizzi M, et al. The edge-to-edge technique: a simplified method to correct mitral insufficiency. Eur J Cardiothorac Surg 1998; 13:240–5.
17. Maisano F, Schreuder JJ, Oppizzi M, et al. The double orifice technique as a standardized approach to treat mitral regurgitation due to severe myxomatous disease: surgical technique. Eur J Cardiothorac Surg 2000;17:201–15.
18. Maisano F, Caldarola A, Blasio A, et al. Midterm results of edge-to-edge mitral valve repair without annuloplasty. J Thorac Cardiovasc Surg 2003; 126(6):1987–97.
19. Maisano F, Vigano G, Calabrese C, et al. Quality of life of elderly patients following valve surgery for chronic organic mitral regurgitation. Eur J Cardiothorac Surg 2009;36(2):261–6.
20. St Goar FG, Fann JI, Komtebedde J, et al. Endovascular edge-to-edge mitral valve repair: short-term results in a porcine model. Circulation 2003;108(16): 1990–3.
21. Condado JA, Acquatella H, Rodriguez L, et al. Percutaneous edge-to-edge mitral valve repair: 2-year follow-up in the first human case. Catheter Cardiovasc Interv 2006;67(2):323–5.
22. Feldman T, Wasserman HS, Herrmann HC, et al. Percutaneous mitral valve repair using the edge-to-edge technique: six-month results of the EVEREST Phase I Clinical Trial. J Am Coll Cardiol 2005; 46(11):2134–40.
23. Feldman T, Kar S, Rinaldi M, et al, EVEREST Investigators. Percutaneous mitral repair with the MitraClip system: safety and midterm durability in the initial EVEREST (Endovascular Valve Edge-to-Edge REpair Study) cohort. J Am Coll Cardiol 2009;54: 686–94.
24. Siegel RJ, Biner S, Rafique AM, et al, EVEREST Investigators. The acute hemodynamic effects of MitraClip therapy. J Am Coll Cardiol 2011;57:1658–65.
25. Naqvi TZ, Buchbinder M, Zarbatany D, et al. Beating-heart percutaneous mitral valve repair using a transcatheter endovascular suturing device in an animal model. Catheter Cardiovasc Interv 2007; 69(4):525–31.

26. Maniu CV, Patel JB, Reuter DG, et al. Acute and chronic reduction of functional mitral regurgitation in experimental heart failure by percutaneous mitral annuloplasty. J Am Coll Cardiol 2004;44(8):1652–61.

27. Siminiak T, Hoppe UC, Schofer J, et al. Effectiveness and safety of percutaneous coronary sinus-based mitral valve repair in patients with dilated cardiomyopathy (from the AMADEUS trial). Am J Cardiol 2009;104(4):565–70.

28. Webb JG, Harnek J, Munt BI, et al. Percutaneous transvenous mitral annuloplasty: initial human experience with device implantation in the coronary sinus. Circulation 2006;113(6):851–5.

29. Daimon M, Gillinov A, Liddicoat J, et al. Dynamic change in mitral annular area and motion during percutaneous mitral annuloplasty for ischemic mitral regurgitation: preliminary animal study with real-time 3-dimensional echocardiography. J Am Soc Echocardiogr 2007;20:381–8.

30. Dubreuil O, Basmadjian A, Ducharme A, et al. Percutaneous mitral valve annuloplasty for ischemic mitral regurgitation: first in man experience with a temporary implant. Catheter Cardiovasc Interv 2007;69(7):1053–61.

31. Sack S, Kahlert P, Bilodeau L, et al. Percutaneous transvenous mitral annuloplasty: initial human experience with a novel coronary sinus implant device. Circ Cardiovasc Interv 2009;2:277–84.

32. Liddicoat JR, Mac Neill BD, Gillinov AM, et al. Percutaneous mitral valve repair: a feasibility study in an ovine model of acute ischemic mitral regurgitation. Catheter Cardiovasc Interv 2003;60(3):410–6.

33. Sack S, Kahlert P, Bilodeau L, et al. Initial human experiences with a non-stented coronary sinus device for the treatment of functional mitral regurgitation in heart failure patients. Circulation 2008;118:S808–9.

34. Aybek T, Risteski P, Miskovic A, et al. Seven years' experience with suture annuloplasty for mitral valve repair. J Thorac Cardiovasc Surg 2006;131(1):99–106.

35. Heuser RR, Witzel T, Dickens D, et al. Percutaneous treatment for mitral regurgitation: the QuantumCor system. J Interv Cardiol 2008;21(2):178–82.

36. Rogers JH, Macoviak JA, Rahdert DA, et al. Percutaneous septal sinus shortening: a novel procedure for the treatment of functional mitral regurgitation. Circulation 2006;113(19):2329–34.

37. Palacios IF, Condado JA, Brandi S, et al. Safety and feasibility of acute percutaneous septal sinus shortening: first-in-human experience. Catheter Cardiovasc Interv 2007;69(4):513–8.

38. Pedersen WR, Block P, Leon M, et al. iCoapsys mitral valve repair system: percutaneous implantation in an animal model. Catheter Cardiovasc Interv 2008;72(1):125–31.

39. Jindani A, Neville EM, Venn G, et al. Paraprosthetic leak: a complication of cardiac valve replacement. J Cardiovasc Surg 1991;32(4):503–8.

40. Safi AM, Kwan T, Afflu E, et al. Paravalvular regurgitation: a rare complication following valve replacement surgery. Angiology 2000;51(6):479–87.

41. Echevarria JR, Bernal JM, Rabasa JM, et al. Reoperation for bioprosthetic valve dysfunction. A decade of clinical experience. Eur J Cardiothorac Surg 1991;5(10):523–6 [discussion: 527].

42. Pate GE, Al Zubaidi A, Chandavimol M, et al. Percutaneous closure of prosthetic paravalvular leaks: case series and review. Catheter Cardiovasc Interv 2006;68(4):528–33.

43. Kort HW, Sharkey AM, Balzer DT. Novel use of the Amplatzer duct occluder to close perivalvar leak involving a prosthetic mitral valve. Catheter Cardiovasc Interv 2004;61(4):548–51.

44. Webb JG, Pate GE, Munt BI. Percutaneous closure of an aortic prosthetic paravalvular leak with an Amplatzer duct occluder. Catheter Cardiovasc Interv 2005;65(1):69–72.

45. Johri AM, Yared K, Durst R, et al. Three-dimensional echocardiography-guided repair of severe paravalvular regurgitation in a bioprosthetic and mechanical mitral valve. Eur J Echocardiogr 2009;10(4):572–5.

46. Messas E, Guerrero JL, Handschumacher MD, et al. Chordal cutting: a new therapeutic approach for ischemic mitral regurgitation. Circulation 2001;104:1958–63.

47. Maisano F, Michev I, Vigano G, et al. Transapical mitral valve repair: chordal implantation with a suction and suture device. Am J Cardiol 2008;102(abstract suppl):8i.

Percutaneous Therapies in the Treatment of Valvular Pulmonary Stenosis

Ronan Margey, MD, MRCPI[a],*, Ignacio Inglessis-Azuaje, MD[b]

KEYWORDS

- Pulmonary stenosis
- Right ventricular outflow tract obstruction
- Balloon pulmonary valvuloplasty • Pulmonic insufficiency
- Percutaneous pulmonary valve replacement

Although obstruction of the right ventricular outflow tract (RVOT) has a number of causes, 80% to 90% of cases are caused by valvular pulmonary stenosis (PS). Isolated PS occurs in 7% to 12% of all congenital heart defects. In most cases, the valve has a classic dome-shaped appearance because of fusion of the valve commissures such that leaflet tip opening is restricted while the leaflet base remains normally mobile.[1,2]

Since the early 1980s, transcatheter balloon pulmonary valvuloplasty (BPV) has become the standard of care in managing symptomatic patients with moderate-to-severe pulmonary valvular stenosis, or asymptomatic patients with severe pulmonary valvular stenosis or with moderate PS and evidence of objective exercise intolerance or right ventricular dysfunction.[3–5] The procedure is safe and complications are rare, with excellent long-term outcomes.

This article discusses the incidence, causes, and pathophysiology of valvular PS in adolescents and adults; its natural history and noninvasive evaluation; the current guideline-recommended indications for BPV; the technical aspects of performing BPV; the immediate and long-term outcomes after valvuloplasty; and the complications and safety of the procedure.

Also discussed is the role of this procedure in neonatal critical PS and in percutaneous pulmonary valve replacement (PPVR) for patients with prior pulmonic valve interventions (valve replacement) or degenerated right ventricle (RV) pulmonary artery (PA) conduits.

OBSTRUCTION OF THE RVOT

Obstruction of the RVOT is congenital or acquired. Congenital obstruction of the RVOT is further subdivided according to the anatomic location of the obstruction into either subinfundibular, infundibular, valvular, or supravalvular obstruction. **Table 1** outlines the differing congenital and acquired causes of obstruction at each respective level.

Subinfundibular obstruction or double-chambered RV is a rare form of RVOT obstruction that results from the division of the RV into an apical hypertrophied high-pressure inlet chamber, and a low-pressure outlet infundibular chamber, separated from each other by a muscular band, the hypertrophied septoparietal trabeculation, and apical shelf, or an abnormal moderator band. The degree of obstruction varies, and is frequently associated with a ventricular septal defect (VSD).[1]

Conflicts of Interest or Financial Disclosures: The authors have nothing to declare.
[a] Structural Heart Disease and Interventional Cardiology, Division of Cardiology, Massachusetts General Hospital and Harvard Medical School, 55 Fruit Street, Boston, MA 02114, USA
[b] Adult Congenital Heart Disease Intervention, Division of Cardiology, Massachusetts General Hospital and Harvard Medical School, 55 Fruit Street, Boston, MA 02114, USA
* Corresponding author.
E-mail address: rmargey@partners.org

Table 1
Types of right ventricular outflow tract obstruction in adults

Category	Level of Obstruction	Causes
Congenital	Subinfundibular	Double-chambered RV (often with VSD)
	Infundibular	Secondary muscular hypertrophy in PS
		ToF
		HOCM (Noonan syndrome)
		Tricuspid valve tissue
		Fibrous tag from IVC/SVC
		Aneurysm of SoV
		Aneurysm of membranous septum
	Valvular	Dome-shaped valve
		Dysplastic valve (Noonan syndrome)
		Unicuspid or bicuspid valve
	Supravalvular	Hourglass deformity at valve
		Pulmonary artery membrane
		Pulmonary artery stenosis
		Peripheral pulmonary artery stenosis
		Associations: congenital rubella; Alagille, Williams, Noonan, and Keutel syndromes
Postoperative	Valvular	Native valve restenosis
		Prosthetic valve restenosis
	Conduit stenosis	
	Peripheral arterial stenosis after prior systemic-pulmonary shunt procedure	

Abbreviations: HOCM, hypetrophic obstructive cardiomyopathy; IVC, inferior vena cava; PS, pulmonary stenosis; RV, right ventricle; SoV, sinus of Valsalva; SVC, superior vena cava; ToF, tetralogy of Fallot; VSD, ventricular septal defect.

Infundibular obstruction most commonly occurs in the setting of muscular hypertrophy caused by valvular PS. However, infundibular obstruction in the absence of valvular PS usually occurs in association with other major congenital heart defects, such as tetralogy of Fallot (ToF), transposition of the great vessels, or with a VSD.[1]

Supravalvular obstruction is uncommonly caused by an hourglass deformity of the pulmonary valve with bottle-shaped sinuses and stenosis occurring at the commissural ridge of the valve. More typically, supravalvular obstruction occurs from main PA or branch PA stenosis. These supravalvular pulmonary arterial stenoses rarely occur in isolation, often arising as part of ToF, or as part of Noonan, Williams, Alagille, Keutel, or congenital rubella syndromes. PA stenosis may also arise after prior surgical banding or systemic–pulmonary arterial shunt procedures. The stenosis may be isolated or multiple in nature, and can range from discrete narrowing to diffuse hypoplasia or occlusion.[1]

Finally, the most common cause of RVOT obstruction arises from disorders at the level of the pulmonary valve itself, as outlined in the next section.

INCIDENCE AND PATHOPHYSIOLOGY OF PS
Valvular PS: Incidence, Syndromic Associations, and Morphology

Valvular PS is usually an isolated lesion, and accounts for 80% to 90% of all RVOT obstruction. It occurs in approximately 7% to 12% of all congenital heart defects. Its inheritance rate is low, ranging from 1.75% to 3.6%.[1,2] There are three distinct morphologic types of valvular PS.

1. Classic or typical "dome-shaped" pulmonary valve, characterized by a narrowed central orifice but a preserved mobile valve mechanism. The orifice can range from pinhole to several millimeters in size, usually central in location, but occasionally eccentric. Rudimentary raphae, which are assumed to represent fused commissures, extend from the cusp tips to a variable distance on the base of the dome-shaped valve, and can range in number from zero to seven; most typical, there are three. Commissures are not readily identifiable. The main pulmonary trunk is pathognomically dilated because of medial wall degeneration, and most frequently the dilatation extends to

involve the left PA, because of the preferential direction of the eccentric jet flow from the stenotic orifice. Calcification, although rare in early life, can occur in adults with typical PS.[2,6]

2. Dysplastic pulmonary valve occurs in approximately 20% of cases. The leaflets are poorly mobile and there is marked myxomatous thickening of the leaflets, with no commissural fusion. Dysplastic PS is frequently seen in patients with Noonan syndrome, an autosomal-dominant disorder with variable penetrance, and in 50% of cases there is a missense mutation in the PTPN II gene on chromosome 12. This syndrome, occurring in 1:1000 to 1:2000 live births, is characterized by characteristic facies, webbed neck, hypotelorism, short stature, and cryptorchidism in males, and hemostatic abnormalities caused by partial factor XI deficiency. Frequently, they also have concomitant infundibular hypertrophy and asymmetric hypertrophy of the left ventricular outflow tract reminiscent of hypertrophic cardiomyopathy.[1,6]

3. Unicuspid or bicuspid pulmonary valve is usually seen in the context of ToF, and may or may not result in PS or regurgitation.[1]

Lastly, postoperative valvular PS can occur as homograft or bioprosthetic pulmonary valve replacements degenerate over time and develop progressive stenosis or regurgitation.

Pathophysiology of Valvular PS

Obstruction of the RVOT at the level of the pulmonary valve results in a rise in RV afterload. In response to this increased afterload, physiologic ventricular muscle hypertrophy occurs, producing thicker chamber walls, decreased compliance, increased ventricular stiffness, and higher right atrial filling pressures.[1,7]

As compliance deteriorates and diastolic dysfunction worsens, venous congestion may occur, initially with exercise but eventually at rest also, limiting cardiac output and the patient's physical activity. This is because, with exercise, pulmonary blood flow is fixed and cannot increase further, resulting in left ventricular preload reductions and limitation of systemic cardiac output.

When obstruction becomes critically severe, substantial increases in RV afterload can lead to systolic failure of the RV, resulting in the clinical symptoms and signs of right heart failure hepatic congestion, jugular venous distention, ascites, and edema. Finally, right ventricular ischemia can also contribute to exercise intolerance. With advanced right ventricular hypertrophy, myocardial oxygen demand increases, and at the same time, the elevated ventricular end-diastolic pressure prevents coronary perfusion of the RV myocardium. In severe cases, this can propagate chest pain, dyspnea, arrhythmia, syncope, and even sudden cardiac death.

PRESENTATION AND NATURAL HISTORY OF PS: DATA FROM THE SECOND NATURAL HISTORY STUDY OF CONGENITAL HEART DISEASE

Most individuals with mild and moderate PS are asymptomatic, with the diagnosis being made incidentally because of auscultation of a cardiac murmur during childhood or adolescence. Data from the Second Natural History study of congenital heart defects have proved that these individuals lead a normal life and have survival similar to the general population. In this longitudinal follow-up study, patients with mild or moderate PS (peak-to-peak transcatheter gradient of <30 or <50 mm Hg) had survival, symptoms, and need for therapy identical to control patients with no PS.[8]

Pulmonic stenosis is rarely progressive when the initial gradients are mild, but moderate PS can progress because of progressive valvular stenosis or reactive infundibular hypertrophy. The current American College of Cardiology/American Heart Association (ACC/AHA) guidelines recommend 5-year echocardiography follow-up for asymptomatic patients with mild PS and 2- to 5-year follow-up echocardiography for asymptomatic patients with moderate PS to detect any progression.[1]

For patients with severe PS, there is a progressive rise in RV filling pressures and a progressive decline in RV diastolic function initially, but ultimately RV systolic function too if the outflow obstruction is not corrected. Data from the Second Natural History study of congenital heart disease showed poor long-term outcomes for individuals with severe PS (peak-to-peak transcatheter gradient of >50 mm Hg) who did not undergo surgical correction. Those individuals with severe PS (gradients >80 mm Hg) who did undergo surgical valvotomy had excellent survival. A total of 97% of 210 patients in this study who underwent pulmonary surgical valvotomy were in New York Heart Association class I at 25 years of follow-up, with some degree of pulmonary regurgitation (PR) seen on echocardiography in 85%. This long-term coexistent PR can contribute to RV volume overload, progressive RV dilatation, and eventual failure if severe.[8]

On the basis of this natural history study, BPV was initially recommended for patients with peak-to-peak transvalvular gradient greater than

50 mm Hg (if cardiac index was normal) detected at cardiac catheterization.[1,9,10]

NONINVASIVE EVALUATION OF PS

In the past, the diagnosis and determination of severity of valvular PS was made on history, physical examination, electrocardiogram, and the peak-to-peak and mean pressure gradients detected from the PA to the RV on invasive cardiac catheterization. Indeed, the initial recommendations of when to perform surgical valvotomy and BPV were made based on hemodynamic gradient severity.[1,2]

In current practice, however, the diagnosis and estimation of lesion severity is virtually always obained noninvasively, using two-dimensional echocardiography with color Doppler and continuous-wave Doppler estimation of valvular stenosis severity. It is the exception that patients must be referred for invasive catheterization to determine the severity of valvular PS, usually only occurring in cases of serial RVOT obstructive lesions (eg, infundibular stenosis along with valvular and main PA stenosis), when the Bernoulli equation assumptions used at echocardiography are inaccurate.[11–13]

This change in modality to determine valvular stenosis severity is reflected in the recently updated ACC/AHA guidelines on adults with congenital heart disease. In 2006, the valvular heart disease guidelines recommended BPV based on transcatheter estimation of peak-to-peak transvalvular gradients. The 2008 updated guidelines on adults with congenital heart disease now use mean and peak instantaneous Doppler gradients to determine stenosis severity and when to perform balloon valvuloplasty.[1]

Peak-to-peak transvalvular gradients measured at cardiac catheterization are not directly comparable, however, with peak or mean instantaneous Doppler pressure gradients measured by echocardiography. It is suggested that peak-to-peak gradient by cardiac catheterization correlates best with mean Doppler (not the peak instantaneous Doppler) gradient, and that the peak instantaneous gradient systematically overestimates the peak-to-peak cardiac catheterization gradient by slightly more than 20 mm Hg.[1,2,12,13] It is important to keep this in mind when comparing the echocardiography gradient-based 2008 ACC/AHA recommendations with the cardiac catheterization-based 2006 ACC/AHA valvular heart disease guideline recommendations.

Echocardiography also provides a wide range of valuable information in planning valvular interventions (Fig. 1A, B). It allows estimation of RV systolic and increasingly RV diastolic function; it allows detection of coexistent congenital defects, such as an atrial septal defect or VSD; it allows for estimation of right ventricular systolic pressures; it allows classification of valvular stenosis severity based on the peak instantaneous transpulmonic pressure gradient (Table 2); and it allows for annulus measurement to guide balloon number and balloon size choice in advance of percutaneous pulmonic valvuloplasty.

Increasingly, cardiac computed tomography or MRI is also being used to help guide intervention and add more information to the data obtained by echocardiography. Both cardiac computer tomography and MRI provide excellent spatial resolution to delineate the anatomy of the RVOT, allowing for detection and evaluation of serial RVOT obstructive lesions (see Fig. 1C, D). Additionally, they both allow for detection of coexistent congenital lesions. More importantly, particularly with cardiac MRI, they allow for exact measurement of RV ejection fraction, RV dimensions and volumes, PA dimensions, valve annulus, and PA dimensions, and they provide basic physiologic estimations of lesion stenosis severity with gradient measurements, regurgitation volume and regurgitant fraction measurement, and isolation of each individual lesion gradient in cases of serial RVOT obstructive lesions.[2,11,14,15]

HISTORY OF AND INDICATIONS FOR PERCUTANEOUS BPV

In 1948, the first surgical pulmonary valve commissurotomy was performed by Sellors.[16] For the next 30 years, surgical valvotomy was the main therapy for severe PS. In 1953, Rubio-Alvarez and coworkers performed the first pulmonary valvuloplasty, using a specially designed catheter, and succeeded in reducing the mean transvalvular gradient from 90 to 30 mm Hg.[17] In 1979, Semb and colleagues[18] reported performing valvuloplasty using a balloon catheter. Similar to the Rashkind technique for creation of an atrial septostomy, valvuloplasty was performed by means of inflating a balloon in the PA and pulling the inflated balloon back into the RV. In 1982, the first real percutaneous balloon valvuloplasty was attempted in an 8-year-old child by Kan and colleagues.[3] Also in 1982, Pepine and colleagues[5] published the first case series of BPV in adults. Subsequently, BPV has become the method of choice in the treatment of classic domed valvular PS in children and adults.

Traditionally, BPV was recommended for classic domed PS patients with a peak-to-peak gradient

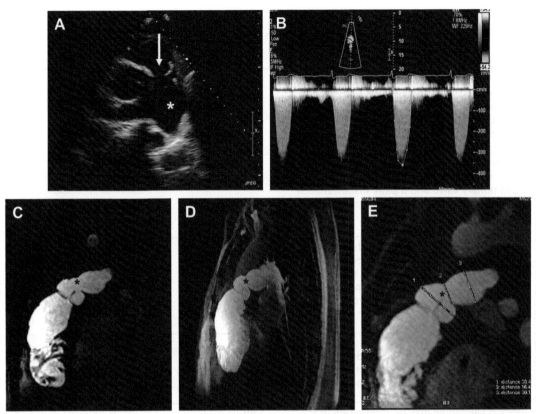

Fig. 1. Noninvasive assessment of pulmonary stenosis. (*A*) Modified short-axis transthoracic echocardiographic view of the RVOT, pulmonary valve, and main PA bifurcation. Note classic doming (*arrow*) of the pulmonary valve leaflets and dilatation of the main and left PA (*asterisk*). (*B*) Continuous wave Doppler of the peak and mean instantaneous transpulmonic valve gradients, measured in this case at 55 and 30 mm Hg, respectively. (*C–E*) Role of cardiac MRI in evaluating anatomy and function before intervention. In this case, a supravalvular stenosis was documented (*asterisk*); maximum diameter stenosis at each of the subvalvular, valvular, and supravalvular levels could be determined. Using phase-contrast cine imaging, it was possible to determine that the RVOT gradient was predominately caused by the supravalvular rather than valvular stenosis.

greater than 50 mm Hg and preserved cardiac index.[2,9,19–21] This recommendation was based on the observation of poor outcome and survival in patients with gradients greater than 50 mm Hg

Table 2
Echocardiographic classification of pulmonary valvular stenosis severity

Severity of Obstruction	Peak Instantaneous Echo Transvalvular Gradient	Right Ventricular Systolic Pressure on Echo
Trivial	<25 mm Hg	<50 mm Hg
Mild	25–49 mm Hg	50–74 mm Hg
Moderate	50–79 mm Hg	75–99 mm Hg
Severe or critical	>80 mm Hg	>100 mm Hg

not treated with surgery in the Second Natural History study of congenital heart disease.[8] The current 2008 ACC/AHA recommendations for management of adult congenital heart disease (**Table 3** for summary) recognize BPV as the first-line treatment for asymptomatic patients with a mean Doppler echocardiography gradient greater than 40 mm Hg and for symptomatic patients with a mean Doppler echocardiography gradient greater than 30 mm Hg (class I recommendation). Additionally, BPV has been considered in patients with moderate stenosis (>30 to <50 mm Hg) in whom there is objective evidence of exercise intolerance or resting or exercise-induced RV dysfunction on cardiopulmonary exercise testing.[1]

Dysplastic valve-related PS was originally considered a contraindication to BPV. However, the current guidelines (see **Table 3**) also endorse BPV in dysplastic valves, for asymptomatic patients with mean Doppler gradients greater

Table 3
Intervention treatment recommendations in patients with valvular pulmonary stenosis

Treatment Recommendation	Class of Recommendation	Level of Evidence
Balloon valvotomy is recommended for asymptomatic patients with a domed pulmonary valve and a peak instantaneous Doppler gradient >60 mm Hg or a mean Doppler gradient >40 mm Hg (in association with less than moderate PR)	I	B
Balloon valvotomy is recommended for symptomatic patients with a domed pulmonary valve and a peak instantaneous Doppler gradient >50 mm Hg or a mean Doppler gradient >30 mm Hg (in association with less than moderate PR)	I	C
Surgical therapy is recommended for patients with severe PS and an associated hypoplastic pulmonary annulus, severe PR, subvalvular PS, or supravalvular PS. Surgery is also preferred for most dysplastic pulmonary valves and when there is associated severe TR or the need for a surgical Maze procedure	I	C
Balloon valvotomy may be reasonable in asymptomatic patients with a dysplastic pulmonary valve and a peak instantaneous Doppler gradient >60 mm Hg or a mean Doppler gradient >40 mm Hg	IIb	C
Balloon valvotomy may be reasonable in selected symptomatic patients with a dysplastic pulmonary valve and a peak instantaneous Doppler gradient >50 mm Hg or a mean Doppler gradient >30 mm Hg	IIb	C
Balloon valvotomy is not recommended for asymptomatic patients with a peak instantaneous Doppler gradient <50 mm Hg in the presence of normal cardiac output	III	C
Balloon valvotomy is not recommended for symptomatic patients with PS and severe PR	III	C
Balloon valvotomy is not recommended for symptomatic patients with a peak instantaneous Doppler gradient <30 mm Hg	III	C

Abbreviations: PR, pulmonary regurgitation; PS, pulmonary stenosis; TR, tricuspid regurgitation.

From Warnes CA, Williams RG, Bashore TM, et al. ACC/AHA 2008 guidelines for the management of adults with congenital heart disease: A report of the American College of Cardiology/American Heart Association task force on practice guidelines (writing committee to develop guidelines on the management of adults with congenital heart disease). Developed in collaboration with the American Society of Echocardiography, Heart Rhythm Society, International Society for Adult Congenital Heart Disease, Society for Cardiovascular Angiography and Interventions, and Society of Thoracic Surgeons. J Am Coll Cardiol 2008;52(23):e1–121; with permission.

than 40 mm Hg, and for symptomatic patients with mean Doppler gradients greater than 30 mm Hg (class II recommendation).[1] Immediate relief of valvular obstruction is less robust when treating dysplastic valve PS, with higher residual mean transvalvular gradients after valvuloplasty described in the Valvuloplasty and Angioplasty of Congenital Anomalies (VACA) registry.[2,12,22–27] Additionally, the long-term success of valvuloplasty in dysplastic valves is more disappointing with higher rates of valvular restenosis. The most important determinant of valvuloplasty success when treating dysplastic valves is the presence of commissural fusion.[2,12,22,23,25–28]

BPV TECHNIQUE
Sedation, Anesthesia, Anticoagulation, Invasive Monitoring, and Antibiotic Prophylaxis

BPV in adults is usually performed under local anesthesia with intravenous conscious sedation using a combination of midazolam and fentanyl. Intramuscular or oral administration of conscious sedation is occasionally used in children undergoing the procedure. General anesthesia with endotracheal intubation is used in infants.

After vascular access is obtained, the patient is typically anticoagulated with intravenous heparin, dosed at 100 units/kg, aiming for an activated clotting time (ACT) of between 200 and 250 seconds. Both anticoagulation and prevention of air entrainment with catheter exchanges are essential in patients with an intracardiac communication (patent foramen ovale, atrial septal defect, or VSD) to prevent possible arterial air embolization or arterial thromboembolic events.

It is the authors' practice to administer a single intravenous dose of antibiotics, usually a third-generation cephalosporin, at the start of the procedure to prevent the potential complication of endocarditis. They use biplane angiography to perform the baseline angiographic and postvalvuloplasty angiography imaging. Finally, continuous heart rate, pulse oximetry, and systemic arterial pressure monitoring should be performed throughout the procedure. Some operators use intracardiac echocardiography to help guide the procedure, although this involves a further femoral venous puncture.[29,30]

Vascular Access

Percutaneous femoral venous access using a modified Seldinger technique is the preferred site of access for pulmonary valvuloplasty.[2] However, other sites of central venous access have been described in the literature, including axillary, jugular, or transhepatic in cases of femoral venous or caval obstruction or occlusion.[2,31,32] Typically a 7Fr or 8Fr catheter 12-cm long sheath is initially placed to perform the baseline right-heart catheterization.

It is the authors' practice to perform right femoral arterial 5Fr catheter access (3 or 4 Fr catheter access in children and adolescents) to continuously monitor arterial blood pressure and systemic oxygenation during the procedure.

Hemodynamic Monitoring and Gradient Assessment

Typical catheters used to perform the hemodynamic assessment are the Berman angiographic catheter or a dual-lumen balloon-wedge catheter (allowing for wire exchanges and pressure measurements). A standard 0.035-in guidewire with a J-tip or a more flexible 0.035-in glidewire (Terumo) or 0.035-in Versacore guidewire can be used to cross the pulmonic valve. If there is difficulty crossing the stenotic valve, the catheter can be exchanged for a multipurpose, Judkins Right, or Cobra catheter and these catheters can be manipulated to cross the valve, after which they can be exchanged for a dual-lumen balloon wedge or dual-lumen pigtail catheter with 5-cm side-holes to allow for simultaneous RV and PA pressure measurement.

Initial baseline right-heart pressure measurements and saturations (to assess for occult intracardiac shunting and calculation of Fick cardiac output) are performed. Measurement of systemic arterial, RV, and PA pressures along with peak-to-peak gradient across the pulmonary valve is performed. This peak-to-peak gradient is used to assess the severity of the pulmonary valve stenosis. Simultaneous RV and femoral arterial pressure is also measured to help evaluate the severity of the pulmonary valve stenosis, with an RV peak systolic pressure greater than 75% of peak systemic systolic pressure considered significant. **Fig. 2** demonstrates peak-to-peak pressure gradients from RV to main PA before and after BPV.

It is not prudent to routinely perform a pullback gradient across the stenotic pulmonic valve especially if it has proved difficult to cross initially. If there are multiple levels of RVOT obstruction then slow pullback from PA bifurcation into the main RV chamber may be required to isolate each individual component of the overall gradient. This can be performed using a dual-lumen catheter with a 0.035-in guidewire or a single-lumen catheter with either an 0.018- or 0.014-in guidewire advanced into the left lower PA preferentially for anchoring while the catheter is slowly withdrawn over the guidewire allowing continuous pressure measurement.

RV Angiography

Biplane RV angiography in anteroposterior (AP; or tilted left anterior oblique 15 degrees and cranial 35 degrees) and lateral views is performed at baseline and after balloon valvuloplasty. The Berman catheter, balloon-wedge catheter, or dual-lumen pigtail catheter can be used to perform the angiography.[2,33] The tip of the catheter is usually withdrawn into the RV apex from where the angiography is performed. This helps to confirm the level of obstruction, evaluate right ventricular chamber

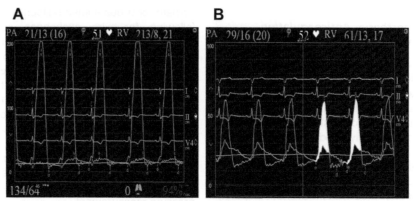

Fig. 2. (*A*) Baseline hemodynamic assessment of severity of pulmonary valvular stenosis. Simultaneous measurement of main PA and RV pressure using a dual-lumen catheter. Note the peak-to-peak gradient of 192 mm Hg. Note also the parvus and tardus waveform on the main PA pressure tracing. Finally, note that the RV systolic pressure is 1.5 times the LV systolic pressure (213 vs 134 mm Hg). (*B*) Post–double BPV hemodynamic assessment. Simultaneous RV and main PA pressure measurements were performed using a dual-lumen catheter. Note the significant change in the pulmonary arterial waveform, with increased waveform amplitude, and marked reduction in the parvus et tardus delay. Note also the reduction in RV systolic pressure from 213 to 61 mm Hg. The peak-to-peak gradient has been reduced to 32 mm Hg after balloon valvuloplasty, with pullback demonstrating much of the residual gradient is occurring below the valvular level because of the infundibular hypertrophy (not shown). This infundibular gradient is seen in up to 30% of cases after BPV and can compromise hemodynamic stability immediately post-BPV. It is best treated by intravenous fluids and β-blockade to improve right ventricular filling.

dimensions and function, and allow pulmonary valve annulus measurement to help guide selection of balloon number and size. A measuring pigtail catheter with 1-cm markers can be used to help measure the annulus size exactly using quantitative coronary angiography software. From the angiographic images, it is possible to appreciate significant infundibular hypertrophy, helping the operator to identify in advance that the patient could develop hypotension or so-called "suicide RV" after balloon valvuloplasty.[34,35] **Fig. 3** demonstrates the typical AP and lateral angiographic images seen in classic dome-shaped pulmonic valve obstruction.

In patients more than 50 years of age with coronary heart disease risk factors, diagnostic coronary arteriography may be performed to exclude significant coronary artery disease.

Preparation for and Performance of Balloon Valvuloplasty

After the baseline hemodynamic evaluation and angiography have been performed, the diagnostic

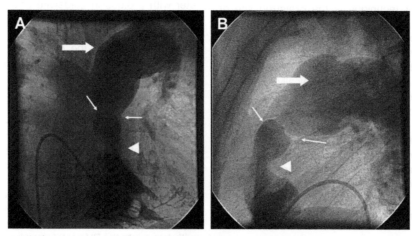

Fig. 3. Right ventricular cineangiography. (*A*) An AP 0-degree, cranial 20-degree projection. (*B*) Lateral projection. Note the classic doming of the pulmonary valve leaflets (*thin arrows*), the poststenotic dilatation preferentially affecting the main and left PA (*thick arrows*), and the infundibular hypertrophy in the RVOT (*arrowheads*).

catheter is readvanced into the main PA, or if a dual-lumen catheter was used initially, the catheter is advanced through the main PA into the left PA, preferably the left lower PA branch. This location ensures excellent stability and anchoring for transitioning the balloon catheters across the pulmonary valve annulus. In neonates and infants undergoing the procedure, a patent ductus arteriosus can be crossed with the guidewire; subsequently, the catheter can be advanced into the descending aorta for stability.[36]

When the initial catheter is in place in the distal left lower PA, an extra stiff support 0.035-in guidewire (Amplatz extra-stiff or super-stiff guidewire) can be advanced into the distal left lower PA. If a double-balloon technique is to be used, a second guidewire can be advanced through the second working channel of the dual-lumen catheter into the distal left lower PA. The catheter is then exchanged and the femoral venous sheath upsized to the required size (usually 12Fr catheter) in single-balloon valvuloplasty or the dilatation balloon catheter can be introduced directly over the guidewire in the case of double-balloon valvuloplasty or if the Inoue balloon is used.

The balloon catheter is then advanced through the right-heart chambers under fluoroscopy across the pulmonary valve annulus. Bony landmarks, valvular calcification, and reference frame imaging are useful tools for positioning the balloon catheter in the ideal location for valvuloplasty.

The balloon is inflated with radiopaque contrast material, diluted 1:4 with sterile saline. In adults undergoing BPV, hand-inflation of the large-caliber balloon catheter is performed; in younger neonates and children, an insufflator device is used to increase the smaller balloon (3–6 mm in diameter) catheter pressure to manufacturer-recommended pressure or until the balloon waist disappears. Optimal balloon inflation is achieved if the waisting of the balloon catheter is totally obliterated. Usually this requires one to two inflation attempts.

As the balloon is inflated, especially in severely stenotic valves, there is a tendency for the balloon to prolapse forward ("melon-seeding"). This can result in suboptimal valve dilatation and iatrogenic main PA injury (dissection or rupture). The balloon can be stabilized in position by many techniques. First, a long introducer sheath can be advanced into the RVOT over the initial support guidewire before the balloon is positioned. Having the sheath located so close to the balloon can aid its stability. Second, gentle backward traction on the balloon catheter shaft as the balloon inflates with simultaneous forward pushing on the guidewire can help to stabilize the balloon across the annulus. Third, placement of the extra-stiff guidewire in a good distal anchoring location can prevent balloon movement. Fourth, longer balloon length can help stabilize the balloon across the annulus as the balloon inflates. Finally, some operators advocate rapid RV pacing (at 180 bpm) or administration of adenosine to produce a sinus pause during balloon inflation to rapidly reduce RV ejection pressure, helping to prevent ejection or prolapsed from the RVOT especially if there is marked baseline infundibular hypertrophy. **Figs. 4** and **5** demonstrate these technical aspects for the double-balloon and single BPV procedures.

Balloon Type, Balloon Diameter, Balloon Length, and Balloon Number

Since the first BPV was performed, the design and engineering of the balloon catheters has significantly evolved, with improvements in the sheath size required, balloon profile, and balloon performance. There are many commercially available balloon catheters available for use in pulmonary valvuloplasty ranging from XXL, Diamond, and Ultrathin (Boston Scientific, Natick, MA, USA); Maxi LD, Opta Pro, and Power flex (Cordis Endovascular, Warren, NJ, USA); and the Tyshak II, Tyshak X, Z-Med II, Z-Med X, and Mullins X (NuMed, Hopkinton, NY, USA).

In the initial recommendations on performing BPV, balloon diameters 1.2 to 1.4 times the valve annulus diameter were recommended. The pulmonary valve annulus is elastic, and it has been established that immediate and longer-term gradient reductions were better with balloons up to 1.4 times the annulus size.[9,22,25,37–43] Balloons greater than 1.5 times the annulus size are not recommended because of the risk of RVOT injury or residual pulmonary insufficiency. However, when performing dysplastic pulmonic valvuloplasty, balloons 1.4 to 1.5 times the annulus dimensions are used. There are increasing concerns regarding the deleterious consequences of PR on long-term RV function and survival, and therefore in recent years there has been a trend to recommend balloon-to-annulus ratios closer to 1.2 than 1.4.[22,24,25,44–47]

Longer balloon lengths are used in adult patients, typically 40 mm in length. Shorter balloons, especially with infundibular hypertrophy and hyperdynamic function, can be more challenging to stabilize in position and prevent melon-seeding. It is worthwhile remembering, however, that although the balloon is more stable, the longer wings and body on the balloon can impinge on the tricuspid valve or the conduction system, causing transient complete heart block

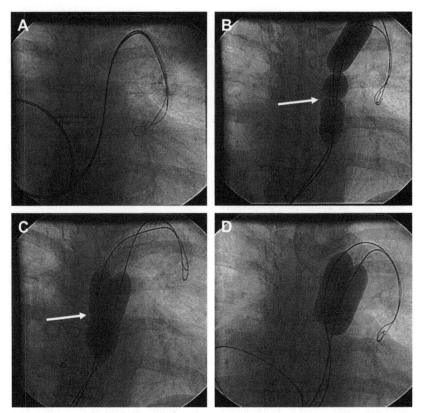

Fig. 4. Double BPV. (*A*) Placement of two 0.035-in extra-stiff Amplatz (Meditech) guidewires through a dual-lumen 8Fr catheter into the left lower PA for support. Note the atrial loop in the catheter to ensure crossing into the RV without entanglement in the tricuspid subvalvular apparatus. (*B*) Significant waisiting (see *white arrow*) on a single balloon inflated at the valve annulus. Note the pulmonary valve stenosis is so severe, that the second balloon melon-seeded forward into the main PA on inflation. (*C*) Typical appearance of double-balloon inflation at the pulmonary valve annulus. Two Z-Med 18 mm × 50 mm balloons were inflated simultaneously. Note the residual waisting on the balloons. The goal of inflation is to see elimination of the waisting on the balloons (see *white arrow*). (*D*) Maximal inflation of both balloons with obliteration of the waisting at the pulmonary annulus.

on inflation. In neonates and infants, and children and adolescents, balloons of 20 and 30 mm length, respectively, are used.

In adults the annulus is frequently too large to dilate with a single balloon. In this situation, double-balloon simultaneous inflation is performed.[7,9,37,42,48–50] When two balloons are used, the following simple formula can be used to calculate the effective balloon size;

$$\text{Effective balloon diameter} = 0.82\,(D1 + D2),$$

where D1 and D2 are the diameters of the balloons used. Although the double-balloon technique produces excellent results, similar to those observed in patients treated with single-balloon inflation, it does involve an extravenous puncture (if dual-lumen catheter is not initially used). There have been case reports of triple BPV for patients with large pulmonary annulus.[33,51]

The Inoue balloon has been used to perform BPV in adults. The major advantage to using this balloon is that the balloon diameter can be incrementally increased by adding extra contrast: saline mixture to the balloon.[2,52,53] There are also many case reports on the use of bifoil or trefoil balloon catheter systems in pulmonary valvuloplasty. The theoretical advantage is purported to be less systemic hypotension during balloon inflation, although these devices are bulky and harder to position than regular balloon catheters.[2,54,55]

Postprocedure and Completion Hemodynamics and Angiography

After valvuloplasty, measurement of the transpulmonic valvular pressure gradient, PA, RV, and systemic arterial pressures, and the pulmonary and systemic oxygen saturation are performed.

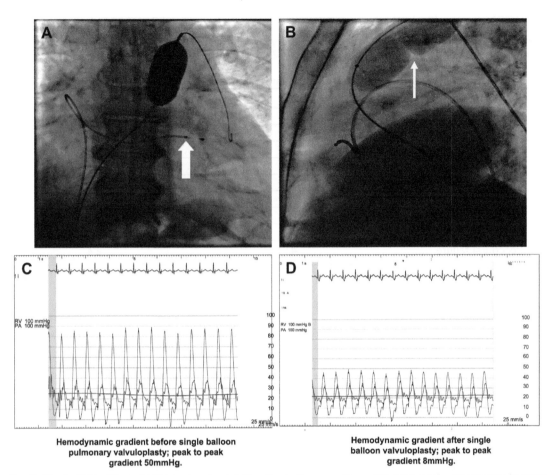

Fig. 5. Single BPV with rapid RV pacing to stabilize the balloon position. (*A*) A 25 mm × 40 mm Cordis Maxi balloon inflated in the AP projection. Note the apparent complete inflation. The *arrow* points to a temporary transvenous pacing wire used to pace the RV at 180 bpm to reduce RV stroke volume acutely to help stabilize the balloon across the pulmonary annulus. (*B*) Lateral projection of the same balloon inflation. Note the importance of the lateral projection in determining if the balloon waist (see *white arrow* of waisting) has been completely ameliorated. In this projection, there is a residual waist seen on the Maxi balloon. (*C*, *D*) Hemodynamic gradients on the single balloon inflation depicted in *A* and *B*. Note the gradient has been reduced from a peak-to-peak of 50 to 8 mm Hg.

The original dual-lumen pigtail catheter or balloon-wedge catheter is readvanced into the main PA to perform the measurement. If a single-lumen catheter is used, then a Tuohy-Borst valve can be used to measure the gradients while maintaining the guidewire position. If there is a significant residual gradient (peak-to-peak valvular gradient >30 mm Hg), then a repeat valvuloplasty can be performed. After satisfactory obliteration of the gradient has been achieved, the Berman or balloon-wedge catheter is advanced back into the RV apex and repeat biplane angiography is performed. Angiography can help assess the leaflet mobility after valvuloplasty and assess for iatrogenic injury, such as flail leaflet, severe PR, tricuspid injury, infundibular stenosis, or PA dissection.

The patients are usually hospitalized overnight after the procedure, with routine monitoring of vital signs and access site monitoring. Patients undergo electrocardiogram and echocardiography on the morning after the procedure. Patients are typically seen with clinical, electrocardiographic, and echocardiography follow-up at 1, 6, and 12 months, and yearly after the procedure.

PROCEDURAL COMPLICATIONS

Complications during or immediately after BPV are rare. In the largest registry of patients undergoing BPV, the VACA registry, the reported death rate was 0.24% and the reported major complication rate was 0.35% in 822 cases.[22] **Table 4** lists the

Table 4
Incidence of complications from balloon pulmonary valvuloplasty in the Valvuloplasty and Angioplasty of Congenital Anomalies registry of 822 cases performed between 1981 and 1986

Incidence of Complication	Number of Cases	% of Total Cases
Children and adults (total 656 procedures)		
Major complications	5	0.8
Minor complications	11	1.7
Incidents	21	3.2
Procedural failure	16	2.4
Infants (total of 168 procedures)		
Major	3	1.8
Minor	8	4.8
Incidents	13	7.7
Procedural failure	4	2.4

complication rates and **Table 5** lists the complication types from the VACA registry.

Bradycardia (or complete heart block if longer balloons are used), ventricular extrasystoles, and systemic hypotension during balloon inflation are typically seen during valvuloplasty. These effects are transient, typically disappearing on balloon deflation.[2,22]

Access site bleeding requiring transfusion although rare has been reported. Other electrophysiologic side effects, such as complete right bundle branch block, bradycardia, and premature ventricular contraction induced R on T polymorphic ventricular tachycardia have been reported.[56,57] Loss of consciousness, cardiac arrest, and cerebrovascular accidents from systemic hypotension after balloon inflation are reported. Balloon injury to the PA (dissection or rupture) and tricuspid valve or papillary muscle injury are very rare.[58–60] Reperfusion pulmonary edema and hemorrhage have been described.[61–63] Cardiac perforation and tamponade has also been reported. Balloon rupture can occur if the recommended burst pressure is exceeded or from eccentric valvular calcification.[2]

The most common complication described in adult patients undergoing BPV is the development

Table 5
Types of complications from balloon pulmonary valvuloplasty in the Valvuloplasty and Angioplasty of Congenital Anomalies registry of 822 cases performed between 1981 and 1986

Types of Complications	Number of Cases	% of Total Cases
Major complications		
Death (one annular tear, one venous tear)	2	0.24
Other (one perforation and tamponade, two tricuspid regurgitation)	3	0.35
Minor complications	(11)	1.34
Venous thrombosis	5	
Venous tears	2	
Respiratory arrest	1	
Leaflet avulsion	1	
Arrhythmia requiring resuscitation	2	
Incidents	(21)	2.55
Arrhythmia (transient)	6	
Hypoxia	3	
Perforation (no tamponade)	1	
Hypotension	1	
Access site bleeding	7	
Arterial thrombosis	2	
Hemoptysis	1	

of severe infundibular obstruction.[64] Infundibular gradients are seen in nearly 30% of cases, with a higher incidence described in the older the patient and more severe the baseline stenosis. This infundibular obstruction can result in the so-called "suicide RV," where the infundibular obstruction prevents adequate left heart filling, producing a downward spiral of systemic hypotension, RV underfilling, and subendocardial RV ischemia that can culminate in circulatory collapse.[34,35,65] If there is a residual infundibular gradient greater than 50 mm Hg after valvuloplasty, then the patient should receive β-blocker therapy along with intravenous fluid boluses to prevent the systemic hypotension.[34] Over time, as the right ventricular hypertrophy regresses, the infundibular obstruction and gradient fades, usually significantly reduced at 6-month follow-up.[66–68]

Femoral venous injuries with deep vein thrombosis or occlusion have been reported, more commonly in infants.[22] Finally, the issues of pulmonary valve restenosis and PR are discussed in greater detail in the next section.

IMMEDIATE AND LONG-TERM RESULTS

Immediately after balloon valvuloplasty there is a decline in the peak-to-peak gradient across the pulmonary valve (see **Figs. 3** and **5**) and a decline in right ventricular systolic pressure. The cardiac index may be unchanged or increase slightly. It is possible on angiography to see improved leaflet mobility and less doming of the leaflets. RV function and tricuspid regurgitation may improve on echocardiography, and if there is an intracardiac shunt, there may be a decrease in right-to-left shunting.[2,69]

BPV is a highly successful procedural with the pooled analysis of 822 patients in the VACA registry demonstrating a clinical success of 98%, with up to 25% having total elimination of transvalvular pressure gradient immediately after the procedure.[1,22] These initial excellent results are maintained in most patients at medium term (2 year) follow-up. However, about 8% to 10% of patients develop restenosis in follow-up.[4,9,12,21,24,25,70–73] Repeat BPV is the treatment of choice for restenosis. In this situation, balloon diameters larger than the initial valvuloplasty are used. In the case of dysplastic valve restenosis, or concomitant supravalvular stenosis, surgery may be the preferred treatment choice for pulmonary valve restenosis.[2,70]

Two risk factors for recurrent valvular stenosis have been identified across several studies: balloon/annulus ratio less than 1.2, and an immediate postvalvuloplasty gradient greater than 30 mm Hg.[2,9,12,13,23–25,27,28,40,41,72,74–79] In addition, the VACA registry identified earlier study year (perhaps indicating operator learning curve), small valve annulus (hypoplastic pulmonary annulus), and complex native or postsurgical PS as predictors of possible restenosis.[24] Other studies have suggested that restenosis is more frequent after balloon valvuloplasty of dysplastic pulmonary valves.[27,70]

Long-term follow-up data to 10 years are now available revealing low residual gradients and minimal late restenosis (<1%), with the need for surgical intervention in approximately 5%. Actuarial freedom from reintervention was 88% and 84%, respectively, at 5 and 10 years.[24,25] In the VACA registry, follow-up data are available on 533 patients at a mean of 8.7 years after valvuloplasty. A suboptimal result (defined as residual gradient >36 mm Hg at the end of the procedure) was present in 23%. Valve morphology and annulus size were the most significant predictors of long-term results. PR was more commonly seen when the balloon/annulus ratio exceeded 1.4. Subjective grades of PR reported were none (26%); trivial (22%); mild (45%); moderate (7%); and severe (0%). More than mild PR was associated with dysplastic valve morphology, small annulus diameter, associated cardiac defects, higher balloon/annulus ratio, and higher immediate postvalvuloplasty gradient.[24,25] Other studies have reported PR of some degree in 40% to 90% of patients after valvuloplasty. The prevalence and severity tends to increase over time. However, it has been traditionally assumed that the clinical consequences are minimal (although recent literature suggests higher RV dysfunction, decreased exercise tolerance, and poor survival in patients with severe PR) and the need for surgical valve replacement is rare (5%).[44,46]

COMPARISON WITH AND ROLE OF SURGERY

No large number multicentered randomized control trial has been performed comparing BPV with surgical valvotomy. However, BPV has lower morbidity and mortality than surgical valvotomy.[2]

There have been several studies comparing balloon valvuloplasty with a matched surgical control cohort.[80–83] O'Connor and colleagues[80] reported on 20 BPV procedures compared with age and gradient-matched surgical controls. In this study, there were slightly higher postprocedure Doppler peak instantaneous gradients in the BPV group (24 ± 2.7 mm Hg) than in the surgical group (16 ± 1.5 mm Hg). There was no PR in 55% of the BPV group, with 45% having mild

PR. However, in the surgical cohort, there was mild PR in 45% and moderate PR in 45%.

Surgery remains an important treatment modality for patients with combined severe PS and PR, recurrent pulmonary valve restenosis, dysplastic pulmonary valves, prior bioprosthetic or homograft stenosis (**Fig. 6**), conduit stenosis resistant to balloon dilatation or stenting, and in patients with multiple levels of RVOT obstruction or concomitant congenital defects requiring surgery.[1]

BPV IN SPECIAL CIRCUMSTANCES: NEONATAL CRITICAL PS AND PPVR

The focus of this article has been BPV in adolescents and adults with PS. However, this therapy is used successfully to relieve RV outflow obstruction allowing RV growth and development, improve systemic oxygenation, increase pulmonary blood flow, and reduce dependency on the ductus arteriosus in neonatal patients with critical PS and an intact ventricular septum, and in neonatal patients with pulmonary atresia and complex congenital heart disease.[36,84–90] A detailed review of the pathophysiology, indications, and technical considerations of the procedure in these patients groups is beyond the scope of this article.

BPV forms an integral part of the evolving technique of PPVR. Transcatheter PPVR provides a less invasive alternative to surgery in patients with right ventricular-to-PA conduit dysfunction (either calcification with stenosis, or regurgitation).

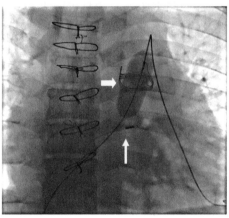

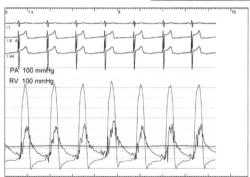

Hemodynamic peak-to-peak gradient from RV (blue) to PA (red), 37mmHg, before BPV.

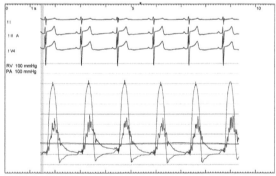

Hemodynamic peak-to-peak gradient from RV (blue) to PA (red), 36mmHg, after BPV.

Fig. 6. Pulmonary valvuloplasty outcomes are not successful for dysplastic valves or prior surgical bioprosthetic valves. This figure shows single BPV of a prior bioprosthetic pulmonary valve replacement using an 18 mm × 40 mm Maxi balloon. The patient had undergone prior open pulmonary valvuloplasty 25 years ago. He subsequently underwent surgical pulmonary valve replacement for free pulmonary regurgitation and RV dilatation 3 years ago with implantation of a bioprosthetic pulmonary valve replacement with an annular dimension of 25 mm. In the 6 months before valvuloplasty, he developed severe exercise intolerance and fatigue, and transthoracic echocardiogram suggested valvular stenosis. The *thick arrow* demonstrates the bioprosthetic valve ring and the *thin arrow* highlights an intracardiac echocardiography catheter used to help guide and image the pulmonary valve intervention. Hemodynamic simultaneous RV (*blue*) to PA (*red*) pressure measurements before and after single BPV show no reduction in the transpulmonic valvular gradient with BPV and the patient underwent redo pulmonic replacement.

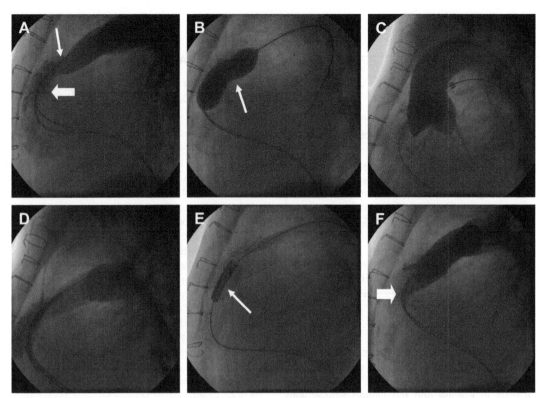

Fig. 7. Percutaneous pulmonary valve replacement using the Melody Ensemble valve replacement system. In this case, a 15 year old with transposition of the great arteries (TGA), VSD, and PA with prior repair and three RV-PA conduit constructions presented with recurrent stenosis and regurgitation at the pulmonic valvular level and RV dilatation. (A) Baseline RVOT cineangiography. Note the dense calcification of the prior RV-PA conduit, greatest at the pulmonic valve level with stenosis (*thin arrow*) and moderate pulmonic insufficiency (*thick arrow*). (B) Balloon angioplasty of the conduit at the level of the existing valve to ensure passage of the valve delivery system into this region. Note the recalcitrant area of stenosis (*arrow*). (C) Aortography, which along with selective coronary angiography allows determination of proximity of pulmonic annulus to the circumflex coronary system and the risk of coronary compression by the Melody valve. (D) Positioning of a balloon expandable stent 20 mm × 36 mm in the RVOT across the prior pulmonic valve. This provides extraradial strength to the Melody valve to prevent recoil and allows full device expansion. It also allows for anchoring of the valve device, which originally only came up to 22 mm in diameter within frequently larger conduits. (E) Tracking of the 22Fr catheter Ensemble delivery system with Melody 22-mm valve (*arrow*) into the previously deployed stent. (F) Deployed valve with PA angiography revealing trace pulmonary regurgitation (*arrow*) caused by the residual wires and catheter passing across the valve leaflets.

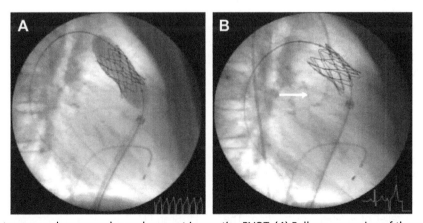

Fig. 8. Percutaneous pulmonary valve replacement in a native RVOT. (A) Balloon expansion of the pulmonic bioprosthesis in the AP cranial projection. To stabilize the valve within the RVOT, the valve expansion is performed under rapid RV temporary transvenous pacing. (B) Expanded stent platform of the pulmonic valve prosthesis in position. Note the Amplatz Left-1 coronary angiographic catheter (*arrow*) being positioned for check coronary angiography after valve deployment.

Box 1
Key Points

1. Pulmonary valvular stenosis is the most common cause of RVOT obstruction.

2. BPV is the treatment of choice for valvular PS.

3. ACC/AHA class Ib recommendation for BPV in patients with asymptomatic severe domed PS (mean gradient on echo >40 mm Hg); class Ic recommendation in patients with symptomatic domed PS (mean gradient on echo >30 mm Hg).

4. Balloon valvuloplasty is a safe and effective therapy, with excellent immediate and long-term relief of valvular obstruction.

The original implantation in humans, performed in 2002, used a bovine jugular vein valve mounted within a balloon-expandable stent.[91] Several clinical trials in Europe and the United States with the commercially available valve–stent platform (Melody valve; Medtronic, Minneapolis, MN, USA) have demonstrated its efficacy in restoring valve competence and reducing conduit pressure gradients.[92–99] **Figs. 7** and **8** demonstrate cases of PPVR. A detailed discussion of PPVR is beyond the scope of this article, and is discussed elsewhere in this issue.

CASE HISTORIES

Four case histories are illustrated by video supplements to this article available in the online version of this article at http://www.cardiology.theclinics.com (Appendix 1). Case 1 (video 1) shows a double BPV. Case 2 is a single BPV with rapid RV pacing (video 2). Case 3 shows complications after pulmonic valvuloplasty, a flail leaflet with moderate PR (video 3). Case 4 is a PPVR (video 4).

SUMMARY

Since its initial introduction in 1982, BPV has been rapidly and widely adopted. BPV is the treatment of choice for pulmonary valve stenosis, representing a safe and effective therapy for the immediate and long-term relief of valvular obstruction. The role of BPV in PPVR continues to be defined and further long-term follow-up studies to determine the significance of residual PR are required. **Box 1** summarizes the key points of this article.

SUPPLEMENTARY DATA

Supplementary data related to this article is found online at doi:10.1016/j.iccl.2011.12.001.

REFERENCES

1. Warnes CA, Williams RG, Bashore TM, et al. ACC/AHA 2008 guidelines for the management of adults with congenital heart disease: A report of the American College of Cardiology/American Heart Association task force on practice guidelines (writing committee to develop guidelines on the management of adults with congenital heart disease). Developed in collaboration with the American Society of Echocardiography, Heart Rhythm Society, International Society for Adult Congenital Heart Disease, Society for Cardiovascular Angiography and Interventions, and Society of Thoracic Surgeons. J Am Coll Cardiol 2008;52(23):e1–121.

2. Rao PS. Percutaneous balloon pulmonary valvuloplasty: state of the art. Catheter Cardiovasc Interv 2007;69(5):747–63.

3. Kan JS, White RI Jr, Mitchell SE, et al. Percutaneous balloon valvuloplasty: a new method for treating congenital pulmonary-valve stenosis. N Engl J Med 1982;307(9):540–2.

4. Kan JS, White RI Jr, Mitchell SE, et al. Percutaneous transluminal balloon valvuloplasty for pulmonary valve stenosis. Circulation 1984;69(3):554–60.

5. Pepine CJ, Gessner IH, Feldman RL. Percutaneous balloon valvuloplasty for pulmonic valve stenosis in the adult. Am J Cardiol 1982;50(6):1442–5.

6. Benson LN, Smallhorn JS, Freedom RM, et al. Pulmonary valve morphology after balloon dilatation of pulmonary valve stenosis. Cathet Cardiovasc Diagn 1985;11(2):161–6.

7. Kern MJ, Bach RG. Hemodynamic rounds series II: pulmonic balloon valvuloplasty. Cathet Cardiovasc Diagn 1998;44(2):227–34.

8. Hayes CJ, Gersony WM, Driscoll DJ, et al. Second natural history study of congenital heart defects. Results of treatment of patients with pulmonary valvar stenosis. Circulation 1993;87(Suppl 2): I28–37.

9. Herrmann HC, Hill JA, Krol J, et al. Effectiveness of percutaneous balloon valvuloplasty in adults with pulmonic valve stenosis. Am J Cardiol 1991;68(10):1111–3.

10. Sherman W, Hershman R, Alexopoulos D, et al. Pulmonic balloon valvuloplasty in adults. Am Heart J 1990;119(1):186–90.

11. Shah PM. Tricuspid and pulmonary valve disease evaluation and management. Rev Esp Cardiol 2010;63(11):1349–65.

12. Marantz PM, Huhta JC, Mullins CE, et al. Results of balloon valvuloplasty in typical and dysplastic

pulmonary valve stenosis: Doppler echocardiographic follow-up. J Am Coll Cardiol 1988;12(2):476–9.

13. Mullins CE, Ludomirsky A, O'Laughlin MP, et al. Balloon valvuloplasty for pulmonic valve stenosis–two-year follow-up: hemodynamic and Doppler evaluation. Cathet Cardiovasc Diagn 1988;14(2):76–81.

14. Jassal DS, Thakrar A, Schaffer SA, et al. Percutaneous balloon valvuloplasty for pulmonic stenosis: the role of multimodality imaging. Echocardiography 2008;25(2):231–5.

15. Rao PS. Balloon pulmonary valvuloplasty in children. J Invasive Cardiol 2005;17(6):323–5.

16. Sellors TH. Surgery of pulmonary stenosis: a case in which the pulmonary valve was successfully divided. Lancet 1948;1(6513):988.

17. Rubio-Alvarez V, Limon R, Soni J. Intracardiac valvulotomy by means of a catheter. Arch Inst Cardiol Mex 1953;23(2):183–92.

18. Semb BK, Tjonneland S, Stake G, et al. "Balloon valvulotomy" of congenital pulmonary valve stenosis with tricuspid valve insufficiency. Cardiovasc Radiol 1979;2(4):239–41.

19. Chow WH, Chow TC. Percutaneous pulmonary balloon valvuloplasty in adults. Am J Cardiol 1992;69(12):1111–2.

20. Fedderly RT, Beekman RH III. Balloon valvuloplasty for pulmonary valve stenosis. J Interv Cardiol 1995;8(5):451–61.

21. Jaing TL, Hwang B, Lu JH, et al. Percutaneous balloon valvuloplasty in severe pulmonary valvular stenosis. Angiology 1995;46(6):503–9.

22. Stanger P, Cassidy SC, Girod DA, et al. Balloon pulmonary valvuloplasty: results of the valvuloplasty and angioplasty of congenital anomalies registry. Am J Cardiol 1990;65(11):775–83.

23. Rao PS. Balloon dilatation in infants and children with dysplastic pulmonary valves: short-term and intermediate-term results. Am Heart J 1988;116(5 Pt 1):1168–73.

24. McCrindle BW. Independent predictors of long-term results after balloon pulmonary valvuloplasty. Valvuloplasty and Angioplasty of Congenital Anomalies (VACA) registry investigators. Circulation 1994;89(4):1751–9.

25. McCrindle BW, Kan JS. Long-term results after balloon pulmonary valvuloplasty. Circulation 1991;83(6):1915–22.

26. David SW, Goussous YM, Harbi N, et al. Management of typical and dysplastic pulmonic stenosis, uncomplicated or associated with complex intracardiac defects, in juveniles and adults: use of percutaneous balloon pulmonary valvuloplasty with eight-month hemodynamic follow-up. Cathet Cardiovasc Diagn 1993;29(2):105–12.

27. Ballerini L, Mullins CE, Cifarelli A, et al. Percutaneous balloon valvuloplasty of pulmonary valve stenosis, dysplasia, and residual stenosis after surgical valvotomy for pulmonary atresia with intact ventricular septum: long-term results. Cathet Cardiovasc Diagn 1990;19(3):165–9.

28. Rao PS, Fawzy ME, Solymar L, et al. Long-term results of balloon pulmonary valvuloplasty of valvar pulmonic stenosis. Am Heart J 1988;115(6):1291–6.

29. Chessa M, Butera G, Carminati M. Intracardiac echocardiography during percutaneous pulmonary valve replacement. Eur Heart J 2008;29(23):2908.

30. Follman DF, Levin TN, Lang RM, et al. Low-frequency intracardiac ultrasonographic imaging before and after balloon pulmonary valvuloplasty. Am Heart J 1993;125(1):259–62.

31. Chaara A, Zniber L, el Haitem N, et al. Percutaneous balloon valvuloplasty via the right internal jugular vein for valvular pulmonic stenosis with severe right ventricular failure. Am Heart J 1989;117(3):684–5.

32. Joseph G, Kumar KP, George PV, et al. Right internal jugular vein approach as an alternative in balloon pulmonary valvuloplasty. Catheter Cardiovasc Interv 1999;46(4):425–9.

33. van den Berg EJ, Niemeyer MG, Plokker TW, et al. New triple-lumen balloon catheter for percutaneous (pulmonary) valvuloplasty. Cathet Cardiovasc Diagn 1986;12(5):352–6.

34. Thapar MK, Rao PS. Use of propranolol for severe dynamic infundibular obstruction prior to balloon pulmonary valvuloplasty (a brief communication). Cathet Cardiovasc Diagn 1990;19(4):240–1.

35. Thapar MK, Rao PS. Significance of infundibular obstruction following balloon valvuloplasty for valvar pulmonic stenosis. Am Heart J 1989;118(1):99–103.

36. Latson L, Cheatham J, Froemming S, et al. Transductal guidewire "rail" for balloon valvuloplasty in neonates with isolated critical pulmonary valve stenosis or atresia. Am J Cardiol 1994;73(9):713–4.

37. Ali Khan MA, Yousef SA, Mullins CE. Percutaneous transluminal balloon pulmonary valvuloplasty for the relief of pulmonary valve stenosis with special reference to double-balloon technique. Am Heart J 1986;112(1):158–66.

38. Cheng TO. Effect of the balloon-to-anulus ratio on pulmonary balloon valvuloplasty. Cardiology 1998;89(2):162.

39. Cheng TO. Percutaneous balloon valvuloplasty for pulmonic stenosis. Cathet Cardiovasc Diagn 1996;39(3):244–5.

40. Mendelsohn AM, Banerjee A, Meyer RA, et al. Predictors of successful pulmonary balloon valvuloplasty: 10-year experience. Cathet Cardiovasc Diagn 1996;39(3):236–43.

41. Narang R, Das G, Dev V, et al. Effect of the balloon-anulus ratio on the intermediate and follow-up results of pulmonary balloon valvuloplasty. Cardiology 1997;88(3):271–6.

42. Rao PS. How big a balloon and how many balloons for pulmonary valvuloplasty? Am Heart J 1988; 116(2 Pt 1):577–80.

43. Rao PS, Thapar MK, Kutayli F. Causes of restenosis after balloon valvuloplasty for valvular pulmonary stenosis. Am J Cardiol 1988;62(13):979–82.

44. Harrild DM, Powell AJ, Tran TX, et al. Long-term pulmonary regurgitation following balloon valvuloplasty for pulmonary stenosis risk factors and relationship to exercise capacity and ventricular volume and function. J Am Coll Cardiol 2010; 55(10):1041–7.

45. Latson LA. Balloon pulmonary valvuloplasty, pulmonary regurgitation, and exercise capacity the good, the bad, and the not yet clear. J Am Coll Cardiol 2010;55(10):1048–9.

46. Bouzas B, Kilner PJ, Gatzoulis MA. Pulmonary regurgitation: not a benign lesion. Eur Heart J 2005;26(5): 433–9.

47. Ammash NM, Dearani JA, Burkhart HM, et al. Pulmonary regurgitation after tetralogy of Fallot repair: clinical features, sequelae, and timing of pulmonary valve replacement. Congenit Heart Dis 2007;2(6): 386–403.

48. Pedra CA, Arrieta SR, Esteves CA, et al. Double balloon pulmonary valvuloplasty: multi-track system versus conventional technique. Catheter Cardiovasc Interv 2006;68(2):193–8.

49. Park JH, Yoon YS, Yeon KM, et al. Percutaneous pulmonary valvuloplasty with a double-balloon technique. Radiology 1987;164(3):715–8.

50. Lau KW, Hung JS. Controversies in percutaneous balloon pulmonary valvuloplasty: timing, patient selection and technique. J Heart Valve Dis 1993; 2(3):321–5.

51. Escalera RB II, Chase TJ, Owada CY. Triple-balloon pulmonary valvuloplasty: an advantageous technique for percutaneous repair of pulmonary valve stenosis in the large pediatric and adult patients. Catheter Cardiovasc Interv 2005;66(3):446–51.

52. Lau KW, Hung JS, Wu JJ, et al. Pulmonary valvuloplasty in adults using the Inoue balloon catheter. Cathet Cardiovasc Diagn 1993;29(2):99–104.

53. Bahl VK, Chandra S, Wasir HS. Pulmonary valvuloplasty using Inoue balloon catheter. Int J Cardiol 1994;45(2):141–3.

54. Meier B, Friedli B, Oberhaensli I, et al. Trefoil balloon for percutaneous valvuloplasty. Cathet Cardiovasc Diagn 1986;12(4):277–81.

55. Thanopoulos BD, Margetakis A, Papadopoulos G, et al. Valvuloplasty with large trefoil balloons for the treatment of congenital pulmonary stenosis. Acta Paediatr Scand 1989;78(5):742–6.

56. Hamaoka K, Sakata K, Onouchi Z. Right ventricular conduction disturbance after balloon valvuloplasty in congenital pulmonary valve stenosis. Lancet 1991;338(8778):1339–40.

57. Steinberg C, Levin AR, Engle MA. Transient complete heart block following percutaneous balloon pulmonary valvuloplasty: treatment with systemic corticosteroids. Pediatr Cardiol 1992;13(3):181–3.

58. Janus B, Krol-Jawien W, Demkow M, et al. Pulmonary artery dissection: a rare complication of pulmonary balloon valvuloplasty diagnosed 11 years after the procedure. J Am Soc Echocardiogr 2006;19(9): 1191.

59. Li Q, Wang A, Li D, et al. Images in cardiovascular medicine. dissecting aneurysm of the main pulmonary artery: a rare complication of pulmonary balloon valvuloplasty diagnosed 1 month after the procedure. Circulation 2009;119(5):761–3.

60. Rohn V, Slais M, Vondracek V. Symptomatic severe tricuspid insufficiency as a late complication of pulmonary balloon valvuloplasty. Prague Med Rep 2010;111(3):235–8.

61. Walker CP, Bateman CJ, Rigby ML, et al. Acute pulmonary edema after percutaneous balloon valvuloplasty for pulmonary valve stenosis. J Cardiothorac Vasc Anesth 2001;15(4):480–2.

62. Cheng TO. Acute pulmonary edema complicating percutaneous balloon valvuloplasty for pulmonic stenosis. J Cardiothorac Vasc Anesth 2002;16(3):391.

63. Cheng HI, Lee PC, Hwang B, et al. Acute pulmonary reperfusion hemorrhage: a rare complication after oversized percutaneous balloon valvuloplasty for pulmonary valve stenosis. J Chin Med Assoc 2009; 72(11):607–10.

64. Ben-Shachar G, Cohen MH, Sivakoff MC, et al. Development of infundibular obstruction after percutaneous pulmonary balloon valvuloplasty. J Am Coll Cardiol 1985;5(3):754–6.

65. Rao PS. Right ventricular filling following balloon pulmonary valvuloplasty. Am Heart J 1992;123(4 Pt 1):1084–6.

66. Fawzy ME, Galal O, Dunn B, et al. Regression of infundibular pulmonary stenosis after successful balloon pulmonary valvuloplasty in adults. Cathet Cardiovasc Diagn 1990;21(2):77–81.

67. Fawzy ME, Hassan W, Fadel BM, et al. Long-term results (up to 17 years) of pulmonary balloon valvuloplasty in adults and its effects on concomitant severe infundibular stenosis and tricuspid regurgitation. Am Heart J 2007;153(3):433–8.

68. Fontes VF, Esteves CA, Sousa JE, et al. Regression of infundibular hypertrophy after pulmonary valvuloplasty for pulmonic stenosis. Am J Cardiol 1988; 62(13):977–9.

69. Carter JE Jr, Feldman T, Carroll JD. Sustained reversal of right-to-left atrial septal defect flow after pulmonic valvuloplasty in an adult. Eur Heart J 1994;15(4):575–6.

70. Ali Khan MA, al-Yousef S, Moore JW, et al. Results of repeat percutaneous balloon valvuloplasty for pulmonary valvar restenosis. Am Heart J 1990; 120(4):878–81.

71. Jarrar M, Betbout F, Farhat MB, et al. Long-term invasive and noninvasive results of percutaneous balloon pulmonary valvuloplasty in children, adolescents, and adults. Am Heart J 1999;138(5 Pt 1):950–4.

72. Kaul UA, Singh B, Tyagi S, et al. Long-term results after balloon pulmonary valvuloplasty in adults. Am Heart J 1993;126(5):1152–5.

73. Lip GY, Singh SP, de Giovanni J. Percutaneous balloon valvuloplasty for congenital pulmonary valve stenosis in adults. Clin Cardiol 1999;22(11):733–7.

74. Rao PS. Long-term follow-up results after balloon dilatation of pulmonic stenosis, aortic stenosis, and coarctation of the aorta: a review. Prog Cardiovasc Dis 1999;42(1):59–74.

75. Shrivastava S, Kumar RK, Dev V, et al. Determinants of immediate and follow-up results of pulmonary balloon valvuloplasty. Clin Cardiol 1993;16(6):497–502.

76. Sievert H, Kober G, Bussman WD, et al. Long-term results of percutaneous pulmonary valvuloplasty in adults. Eur Heart J 1989;10(8):712–7.

77. Silvilairat S, Pongprot Y, Sittiwangkul R, et al. Factors determining immediate and medium-term results after pulmonary balloon valvuloplasty. J Med Assoc Thai 2006;89(9):1404–11.

78. Masura J, Burch M, Deanfield JE, et al. Five-year follow-up after balloon pulmonary valvuloplasty. J Am Coll Cardiol 1993;21(1):132–6.

79. Melgares R, Prieto JA, Azpitarte J. Success determining factors in percutaneous transluminal balloon valvuloplasty of pulmonary valve stenosis. Eur Heart J 1991;12(1):15–23.

80. O'Connor BK, Beekman RH, Lindauer A, et al. Intermediate-term outcome after pulmonary balloon valvuloplasty: comparison with a matched surgical control group. J Am Coll Cardiol 1992;20(1):169–73.

81. Peterson C, Schilthuis JJ, Dodge-Khatami A, et al. Comparative long-term results of surgery versus balloon valvuloplasty for pulmonary valve stenosis in infants and children. Ann Thorac Surg 2003;76(4):1078–82 [discussion: 1082–3].

82. Smolinsky A, Arav R, Hegesh J, et al. Surgical closed pulmonary valvotomy for critical pulmonary stenosis: implications for the balloon valvuloplasty era. Thorax 1992;47(3):179–83.

83. Earing MG, Connolly HM, Dearani JA, et al. Long-term follow-up of patients after surgical treatment for isolated pulmonary valve stenosis. Mayo Clin Proc 2005;80(7):871–6.

84. Weber HS. Initial and late results after catheter intervention for neonatal critical pulmonary valve stenosis and atresia with intact ventricular septum: a technique in continual evolution. Catheter Cardiovasc Interv 2002;56(3):394–9.

85. Rhodes J, O'Brien S, Patel H, et al. Palliative balloon pulmonary valvuloplasty in tetralogy of Fallot: echocardiographic predictors of successful outcome. J Invasive Cardiol 2000;12(9):448–51.

86. Li S, Chen W, Zhang Y, et al. Hybrid therapy for pulmonary atresia with intact ventricular septum. Ann Thorac Surg 2011;91(5):1467–71.

87. Latson LA. Critical pulmonary stenosis. J Interv Cardiol 2001;14(3):345–50.

88. Cholkraisuwat E, Lertsapcharoen P, Khongphatthanayothin A, et al. Balloon pulmonary valvuloplasty in tetralogy of Fallot: effects on growth of pulmonary annulus and transannular patch. J Med Assoc Thai 2010;93(8):898–902.

89. Gildein HP, Kleinert S, Goh TH, et al. Pulmonary valve annulus grows after balloon dilatation of neonatal critical pulmonary valve stenosis. Am Heart J 1998;136(2):276–80.

90. Aburawi EH, Berg A, Pesonen E. Effects of balloon valvuloplasty on coronary blood flow in neonates with critical pulmonary valve stenosis assessed with transthoracic Doppler echocardiography. J Am Soc Echocardiogr 2009;22(2):165–9.

91. Bonhoeffer P, Boudjemline Y, Qureshi SA, et al. Percutaneous insertion of the pulmonary valve. J Am Coll Cardiol 2002;39(10):1664–9.

92. Zahn EM, Hellenbrand WE, Lock JE, et al. Implantation of the melody transcatheter pulmonary valve in patients with a dysfunctional right ventricular outflow tract conduit early results from the U.S. clinical trial. J Am Coll Cardiol 2009;54(18):1722–9.

93. Lurz P, Coats L, Khambadkone S, et al. Percutaneous pulmonary valve implantation: impact of evolving technology and learning curve on clinical outcome. Circulation 2008;117(15):1964–72.

94. Momenah TS, El Oakley R, Al Najashi K, et al. Extended application of percutaneous pulmonary valve implantation. J Am Coll Cardiol 2009;53(20):1859–63.

95. Nordmeyer J, Coats L, Lurz P, et al. Percutaneous pulmonary valve-in-valve implantation: a successful treatment concept for early device failure. Eur Heart J 2008;29(6):810–5.

96. Nordmeyer J, Khambadkone S, Coats L, et al. Risk stratification, systematic classification, and anticipatory management strategies for stent fracture after percutaneous pulmonary valve implantation. Circulation 2007;115(11):1392–7.

97. Nordmeyer J, Lurz P, Khambadkone S, et al. Pre-stenting with a bare metal stent before percutaneous pulmonary valve implantation: acute and 1-year outcomes. Heart 2011;97(2):118–23.

98. Garay F, Webb J, Hijazi ZM. Percutaneous replacement of pulmonary valve using the Edwards-Cribier percutaneous heart valve: first report in a human patient. Catheter Cardiovasc Interv 2006;67(5):659–62.

99. Gatlin SW, Kim DW, Mahle WT. Cost analysis of percutaneous pulmonary valve replacement. Am J Cardiol 2011;108(4):572–4.

Percutaneous Balloon Valvuloplasty for Aortic Stenosis in Newborns and Children

Damien Kenny, MD*, Ziyad M. Hijazi, MD, MPH

KEYWORDS
- Balloon • Aortic • Valvuloplasty

Congenital valvar aortic stenosis (AS) is a highly variable condition, ranging from mild transvalvar flow disturbances secondary to bicuspid aortic valve to severe valvar stenosis in fetal life with consequences for growth of left heart structures.[1] Variability in clinical presentation is mirrored by huge variability in valve morphology; however, in all cases reduced effective orifice area leads to obstruction to flow, usually resulting from thickening and reduced motion of the valve leaflets.

Although no specific etiologic factor has been identified, strong links with inheritable conditions such as Turner syndrome have been demonstrated.[2] Gene deletions contributing to left heart obstructive lesions have also been described.[3,4] Bicuspid aortic valve is the most common congenital cardiac abnormality, affecting 1% to 1.3% of the population, although fewer than 10% of these patients will require intervention for progressive stenosis or regurgitation before the fifth decade of life.[5] True valvar AS accounts for approximately 5% of congenital heart defects and, depending on the degree of stenosis, may require intervention in childhood.

Clinical presentation usually depends on the severity of the stenosis, with the most severe cases presenting soon after birth with low cardiac output secondary to left ventricular dysfunction. In cases of critical AS, neonates are dependent on right-to-left flow across the arterial duct to maintain systemic perfusion, and closure of the duct may lead to death. In less severe cases, progression of stenosis usually occurs throughout childhood, with 17% of patients from one study requiring intervention at a median age of 10.5 years following diagnosis at a median age of 2 years.[6]

Interventional treatment options consist of open surgical valvotomy or balloon valvuloplasty, with both therapies providing excellent but usually only temporary relief of stenosis. This review focuses on balloon aortic valvuloplasty (BAV) as a therapy for congenital valvar AS in infants and children, focusing on established techniques, outcomes, and future challenges.

EVOLUTION OF BALLOON AORTIC VALVULOPLASTY
Approach

Retrograde from the femoral artery
Balloon valvuloplasty of the aortic valve was first reported in 1984 by Lababidi and colleagues.[7] Twenty-three patients aged 2 to 17 years underwent BAV via a retrograde approach from the femoral artery. Following diagnostic hemodynamic assessment including assessment of cardiac

Disclosure: The authors have no conflict of interest and received no financial support for this study. This is an original article and has not been previously published or submitted to another journal.
Rush Center for Congenital and Structural Heart Disease, Rush University Medical Center, 1653 West Congress Parkway, Chicago, IL 60612, USA
* Corresponding author.
E-mail address: Damien_Kenny@rush.edu

Intervent Cardiol Clin 1 (2012) 121–128
doi:10.1016/j.iccl.2011.09.003

output, pull-back gradient across the aortic valve was performed followed by left ventricular angiogram in the left anterior oblique view. A double-lumen 9F balloon catheter was then advanced over a 0.035-inch (0.889 mm) guide wire across the aortic valve, and the balloon (4 cm in length) was inflated sequentially on 3 separate occasions to a diameter 1 mm less than the aortic valve annulus measured by angiography. During this time the second lumen of the balloon catheter was connected externally to the venous catheter in the right atrium via a Y-connector to provide partial decompression of the left ventricle while the aortic valve was fully occluded. Following valvuloplasty, the pull-back gradient was reassessed and an ascending aortogram was performed to evaluate the degree of aortic regurgitation (AR). The mean pressure gradient fell from 113 ± 48 mm Hg preprocedure to 32 ± 15 mm Hg following valvuloplasty. No femoral artery complications were reported, with an increase in the number of patients with mild AR from 6 before the procedure to 10 afterwards.

Since this initial report, numerous modifications to the approach and the equipment available have been performed with the aim of minimizing damage to the vascular access sites, maximizing balloon stability, and providing the greatest reduction in transvalvar gradient with minimal postprocedural AR.

Carotid arterial approach

The classic approach to the aortic valve has continued to be retrograde from the femoral artery. In older children arterial complications may be less likely, due to larger vessel size; however, compromise of the femoral artery is a significant concern in neonates and small infants. Indeed, in a recent report from a single-center 16-year experience with BAV in 30 neonates and infants with congenital AS, 61% of infants undergoing femoral approach had a vascular complication.[8] Four of these patients required emergency surgery with 2 further patients requiring blood transfusion. Due to these complications, in 2003 this group switched to a carotid arterial approach using arterial cutdown, and has had no subsequent arterial complications. Indeed the carotid approach has been advocated by other investigators, with excellent outcomes.[9,10]

Other approaches

Other approaches described include the umbilical artery in newborns with critical aortic stenosis,[11] the axillary artery approach,[12] and the transvenous antegrade approach.[13,14] Approaching the aortic valve from the femoral vein across the atrial septum was first described for AS in children by Hausdorf and colleagues[13] in 1993. The attractive aspects of this approach include not only avoidance of cannulation of the femoral arteries, but potential for more stable balloon position and less inadvertent damage to the aortic valve. Indeed, when comparing these approaches in neonates with severe AS, Magee and colleagues[14] found that the degree of postprocedural AR, which has been repeatedly proved to be an independent risk factor for earlier surgical intervention, was less with the antegrade (venous) approach. Crossing the aortic valve in the same direction as blood flow may reduce the risk of valve leaflet perforation and leaflet avulsion during balloon inflation, thus limiting some of the major precipitants for significant aortic valve damage during valvuloplasty. However, the approach may be technically challenging and certainly carries a risk of complications. Cardiac perforation during transseptal puncture, left ventricular wall perforation, and damage to the mitral valve have all been reported using this approach in smaller patients.

Balloon Stability

Maneuvers to maximize balloon stability during balloon inflation have also evolved. Cardiac contractility of the left ventricle will naturally propel an inflated balloon toward the aorta, resulting in failure of maximal inflation of the balloon across the site of stenosis. Furthermore, excessive balloon motion during inflation may exacerbate leaflet damage, particularly leaflet avulsion. Early attempts to overcome these challenges included use of extra-stiff guide wires or double balloons.[15,16] In the latter technique, the aortic valve is crossed with two separate balloons from two separate retrograde arterial access sites. The collective balloon to annulus diameter ratio is larger (up to 1.3:1) with this technique than a single balloon, allowing more aggressive dilatation but without fully abolishing outflow from the left ventricle during inflation and therefore promoting balloon stability. The other advantage of this approach is the possibility of using two smaller-diameter balloons rather than one larger balloon, thereby reducing potential trauma to the femoral artery; however, with newer lower-profile balloons, this has become less relevant.

In 1998, de Giovanni and colleagues[17] reported on the use of adenosine to promote cardiac standstill for 13 patients with right or left heart obstructive lesions, 6 of whom had AS. The procedure was safe and provided excellent relief of stenosis; however, the time taken for the drug to achieve asystole ranged from 2.4 to 15.8 seconds while the length of asystole ranged from 2.4 to 10.8

seconds, demonstrating significant variability from patient to patient. Subsequent reports described rapid right ventricular pacing as a controlled means of reducing ventricular stroke volume during balloon inflation. Daehnert and colleagues[18] described use of this technique in 14 of 37 children undergoing BAV in whom balloon stability could not be achieved with initial inflation. Pacing rates were set between 220 and 240 beats per minute, with balloon stability achieved in all patients. This approach has become the most widely accepted means of achieving balloon stability during valvuloplasty, and has been expanded with use during intervention on other left heart obstructive lesions with the aim of reducing systemic blood pressure by at least 50% during balloon inflation.[19] Recent modifications for aortic valvuloplasty have been reported, describing pacing of the left ventricle using the guide wire over which the balloon is advanced, with successful capture in all cases and no cases of sustained arrhythmia.[20]

INDICATIONS FOR BALLOON AORTIC VALVULOPLASTY

The American Heart Association (AHA) recently has published guidelines for BAV for patients with congenital valvar AS.[21] Class I recommendations for isolated AS are shown in **Box 1**.

It is worth noting the caveat within these guidelines that the pressure gradients outlined refer to patients sedated during cardiac catheterization, and that catheter gradients in patients under general anesthesia may be lower.

Unfortunately, the decision to perform cardiac catheterization outside those with critical AS is usually based on gradients estimated by transthoracic

---

Box 1
Class I recommendations for isolated congenital AS

- Newborns with critical AS, who are by definition duct dependent, regardless of the measured gradient across the aortic valve

- Infants and children with depressed ventricular function regardless of the measured gradient across the aortic valve

- Children with a resting peak systolic gradient measured at catheter of ≥50 mm Hg

- Children with a resting peak systolic gradient measured at catheter of ≥40 mm Hg if there are symptoms of angina or syncope or ischemic ST-T–wave changes on electrocardiography at rest or with exercise

---

echocardiography (TTE). Significantly elevated peak instantaneous pressure gradients as estimated by TTE do not always equate to peak-to-peak or simultaneous pressure gradients measured in the catheter laboratory. This scenario arises not infrequently, providing a conundrum for the interventionalist, particularly when the patient is under general anesthesia. Class IIb recommendations from the AHA suggest that aortic valvuloplasty may be considered for asymptomatic patients with a catheter-obtained peak systolic gradient of less than 50 mm Hg when the patient is heavily sedated or anesthetized if a nonsedated Doppler study finds the mean valve gradient to be greater than 50 mm Hg. Clearly this leaves some room for the operator to assimilate all the information at hand and to tailor a decision on whether to intervene or not based on these data. The other scenario is a situation in which inaccurate assessment of the true degree of AS occurs in the setting of reduced ventricular systolic function. The AHA recommendations suggest that BAV should be considered irrespective of the measured gradient across the aortic valve if systolic ventricular dysfunction is present.

THE PROCEDURE

As already discussed, variability in approach to BAV may exist based on operator preference and experience. A consistent approach within each center, however, is advisable. Patient selection is important, particularly in neonates with AS associated with a borderline left ventricle or endocardial fibroelastosis, when despite adequate relief of the transvalvar gradient, the left ventricle may not be sufficient to sustain adequate cardiac output in the longer term. However, growth of the left heart has been demonstrated following aortic valvuloplasty for critical AS, and conversion to a functionally univentricular circulation is still feasible following valvuloplasty.[22]

Neonates, Young Infants, Critically Ill Patients, and Those Requiring a Transcarotid Approach

In the authors' center, in neonates, young infants and critically ill patients, or in those requiring a transcarotid approach, these procedures are performed under general anesthesia. Deep sedation may be considered in older patients undergoing semielective BAV; however, this may need to be tailored to how well it is perceived the child or adolescent will tolerate this approach. In neonates, right carotid cutdown is preferred with placement of a 4F short sheath, and the valve is crossed with a 0.018-inch (0.457 mm) floppy-tipped wire advanced through a 4F Judkins right catheter, performing all catheter and balloon exchanges over this single wire.[23] Valve annulus measurements are estimated from preprocedural TTE, although with the evolution of the micro–transesophageal echocardiography (TEE) probes, TEE may also be feasible to guide the procedure in infants as small as 1.7 kg.[24] Normally a low-profile balloon, such as the Tyshak Mini balloon (NuMED Inc, Hopkinton, NY, USA) is used to dilate the valve. A balloon 2 cm in length and 1 mm less than the measured annular diameter is chosen, as data suggests that balloon to annulus diameters of greater than 1 lead to substantial increases in significant postprocedural AR.[25] Transvalvar gradients following dilatation may be evaluated with a Multitrack Catheter (NuMED Inc) without compromising wire position, and balloon sizes up to the measured annular diameter may be considered if there are persisting significant gradients without significant development of AR. Rapid right ventricular pacing is usually not required for balloon stability in neonates, due to faster heart rates and smaller stroke volumes; however, if chosen, caution is advised because of reports of myocardial perforation with temporary pacing leads.[26]

Older Children

In older children, a retrograde femoral arterial approach is used. The valve is crossed with a 0.035-inch (0.889 mm) straight-tipped guide wire through an AL-1 catheter. In cases where difficulty is encountered crossing the valve, ascending aortic angiography may reveal the stenotic jet and guide valve crossing. Once the valve has been crossed, the guide wire is exchanged for a stiffer 0.035-inch J-tipped wire placed in the left ventricular apex (**Fig. 1**). Similarly, lower-profile balloons, such as the Tyshak II balloon catheter (NuMED Inc), although unable to provide higher inflation pressures, should be sufficient to expand the valve in patients with noncalcific congenital AS. Initial balloon diameters are chosen at approximately 90% of the measured aortic annular diameter, as before. In these older patients, the authors advocate the use of intracardiac echocardiography (ICE) through an 8F sheath in the femoral vein. This procedure provides excellent views of the aortic valve (measurement of the annulus) and allows an online assessment of AR without the need for repeated aortography and potential loss of wire position (**Fig. 2**). Before positioning the balloon catheter, a 5F pacing lead catheter is placed in the apex of the right ventricle and tested to ensure good capture with rate set to achieve a 50% reduction in systolic aortic blood

pressure. Immediate procedural efficacy may be assessed in older patients by measuring simultaneous pressures in the left ventricle and ascending aorta using a double-lumen pigtail catheter, or by measuring peak-to-peak gradient across the aortic valve using a multitrack catheter as previously described. Repeat ascending aortogram may be considered to assess the degree of post-valvuloplasty AR; alternatively, if ICE is used, it can accurately demonstrate the presence (degree) or absence of AR.

PROCEDURAL COMPLICATIONS

Box 2 lists complications of BAV. In the current era, mortality is uncommon with BAV, particularly as surgical options for the borderline left ventricle have evolved over the last 10 years.

Valve Damage

The main concern associated with BAV, irrespective of age, is valve damage leading to significant postprocedural AR. Numerous large follow-up studies, as discussed earlier, have identified development of moderate to severe AR as an independent predictor for earlier surgical reintervention following valvuloplasty.[22,27] The incidence of postvalvuloplasty AR has been reported at approximately 25%,[27,28] with older patients noted to be more often at risk.[27] Avoidance of higher balloon/annulus ratios may reduce the incidence and degree of immediate postprocedural AR[25,29]; however, some reports suggest that progression of AR may occur over time irrespective of the initial balloon size used and may be related to valve morphology.[30] These reports emphasize the fact that despite advances in balloon design and operator experience, it is difficult to predict the response of each individual's valve to valvuloplasty even within recommended balloon/annulus ratios.

Acute Vascular Damage

The other main procedural complication reported with BAV predominantly in neonates and infants is acute vascular damage, particularly femoral arterial compromise. Historically, with larger required sheath sizes, this was reported as high as 45% and included arterial disruption or tear in 38% of this patient group,[31] with a mean age at procedure of 6.4 years. This potential for acute femoral arterial damage has persisted through more contemporary reports as discussed earlier,[8] with chronic effects on the femoral arteries being unknown, although reports suggest that these are not insignificant.[32] Alternative arterial access approaches have been reported with significantly

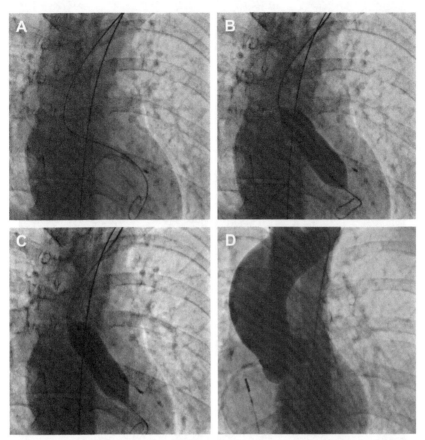

Fig. 1. Series of fluoroscopy images demonstrating approach to balloon aortic valvuloplasty in an adolescent female with valvar aortic stenosis. (*A*) The balloon catheter crosses the aortic valve with the guide wire in the left ventricular apex. The right ventricular pacing lead and the intracardiac echocardiography catheter are also seen within the heart. (*B*) Following initial balloon inflation there is some residual waste; however, this disappears on full inflation (*C*). (*D*) Final aortic angiogram demonstrates no significant aortic incompetence.

lower levels of arterial compromise, and should be considered in younger infants.[10,12]

Other Complications

Other reported complications include thromboembolic events,[33] cardiac arrhythmias including complete heart block,[34] damage to the mitral valve particularly with an antegrade venous approach,[14] and perforation of the ventricular myocardium.[35] Higher complication rates (up to 15%) have been reported in younger infants, and therefore particular care is needed in this patient group.[35]

LONGER-TERM OUTCOMES

Numerous large contemporary retrospective follow-up studies have demonstrated that BAV provides excellent transvalvar gradient relief in infants and children with congenital AS (**Table 1**). However, in the majority of circumstances, reintervention is required with the expectation that

eventual surgical repair or replacement of the valve will be necessary.

In the largest follow-up study in the United States, evaluating 509 patients over a median follow-up of 9.3 years, mean survival free from any aortic valve reintervention at 5 years was 72%, at 10 years 54%, and at 20 years 27%.[27] Just fewer than 50% of patients required an aortic valve replacement at 20 years of follow-up. In multivariate analysis, lower postdilatation gradient and lower grade of AR were associated with longer freedom from aortic valve replacement. However, even mild postprocedural rates of AR were associated with the need for aortic valve replacement, suggesting that AR may worsen with time, as already discussed. This study excluded 54 patients converted to a univentricular circulation or who died 30 days or less after the procedure.

Other reported studies without exclusion criteria as listed below have shown similar survival free from aortic valve surgery. Fratz and colleagues,[28] looking at 188 patients over a 17-year follow-up

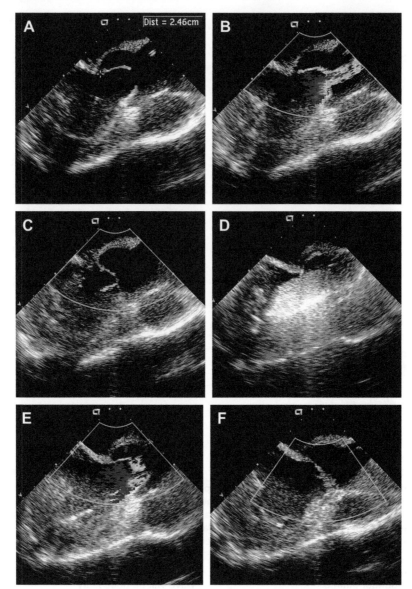

Fig. 2. Series of intracardiac echocardiography images used to guide balloon aortic valvuloplasty in an older child. (*A*) Clear images of the aortic valve are obtained, allowing accurate measurement of the aortic annulus. (*B*) Color Doppler demonstrates turbulent flow across the valve with restricted opening of the valve leaflet tips and (*C*) trivial aortic incompetence. (*D*) Stable balloon position across the aortic valve is seen, with (*E*) improved aortic valve opening and (*F*) no increase in aortic valve regurgitation.

Box 2
Complications of BAV

- Valve damage leading to significant postprocedural AR
- Acute vascular damage, particularly femoral arterial compromise
- Thromboembolic events
- Cardiac arrhythmias including complete heart block
- Damage to the mitral valve, particularly with an antegrade venous approach
- Perforation of the ventricular myocardium

---

period until 2004, evaluated survival free from aortic valve surgery based on age at BAV. Patients undergoing BAV less than 1 month old had a 10-year surgery-free survival of 59%, whereas those older than 1 month demonstrated 70% surgery-free survival. Approximately 10% of patients in each group required a repeat balloon procedure.

In the largest follow-up study to date looking at 1004 patients from multiple European centers, Ewert and colleagues[35] reported a freedom from surgical intervention of approximately 70% at 5 years and 50% at 10 years of follow-up. In this series balloon reinterventions were more common in newborns (16%) than in those outside the

Table 1
Contemporary retrospective follow-up studies of BAV

Authors	Year	No. of Patients	Age at BAV[a]	Gradient Reduction	Freedom from Reintervention
McCrindle et al[36]	2001	82	2 d	69–20 mm Hg	48%, 5 y[b]
Fratz et al[28]	2008	188	8 d, 5.6 y[c]	Refer to published diagram	59% (<1/12) and 70% (>1/12), 10 y (S)
Brown et al[27]	2010	509	2.4 y	Median reduction 35 mm Hg	72%, 5 y; 54%, 10 y; 53%, 20 y
Ewert et al[35]	2011	1004	3.6 mo	65–26 mm Hg	50%, 10 y (S)

(S) indicates surgical reintervention.
[a] Age may indicate either mean or median values.
[b] *Estimated* freedom from reintervention.
[c] Two groups based on age at procedure: <1 month and >1 month.

newborn period (10%). There has only been one significant study evaluating retrospective comparative outcomes in neonates undergoing either surgical valvotomy or balloon valvuloplasty for critical AS. This study looked at follow-up data on 110 neonates over a 5-year period from 1994 to 1999.[36] Higher residual median transvalvar gradients were seen in the surgical group, whereas clinically significant AR was seen more commonly in the group undergoing balloon valvuloplasty. Of note, time-related survival was only 72% at 5 years with no difference between the groups. Independent risk factors for mortality included mechanical ventilation prior to the procedure and smaller aortic valve annulus z score. Estimated freedom from reintervention was 48% at 5 years, again with no difference seen between the groups. This result is somewhat lower than the figures reported in the other studies discussed; however, this report evaluated exclusively neonates with critical AS, suggesting reintervention rates may be higher in this group as indicated by Franz and colleagues.[28] Similar to the report by Ewert and colleagues,[35] this study evaluated data from multiple centers, and this may have influenced the slightly lower freedom from reintervention rates seen with these two studies.

SUMMARY

BAV has evolved into a viable alternative to surgical valvotomy in patients with congenital AS. Immediate and progressive AR may prognosticate the need for surgical reintervention, and aortic valve replacement may be required in this setting. Future endeavors should concentrate on maneuvers to minimize valve damage during balloon inflation to limit the degree of postprocedural regurgitation.

REFERENCES

1. Hornberger LK, Sanders SP, Rein AJ, et al. Left heart obstructive lesions and left ventricular growth in the midtrimester fetus. A longitudinal study. Circulation 1995;92:1531–8.
2. Rainier-Pope CP, Cunningham RD, Nadas AS, et al. Cardiovascular malformation in Turner's syndrome. Pediatrics 1964;33:919–25.
3. Zhao W, Wang J, Shen J, et al. Mutations in VEGFA are associated with congenital left ventricular outflow tract obstruction. Biochem Biophys Res Commun 2010;396:483–8.
4. Garg V, Muth AN, Ransom JF, et al. Mutations in NOTCH1 cause aortic valve disease. Nature 2005;437:270–4.
5. Roberts WC, Ko JM. Frequency of unicuspid, bicuspid and tricuspid aortic valves by decade in adults having aortic valve replacement for isolated aortic stenosis. Circulation 2005;111:920–5.
6. Kitchiner D, Jackson M, Walsh K, et al. The progression of mild congenital aortic valve stenosis from childhood into adult life. Int J Cardiol 1993;42:217–23.
7. Lababidi Z, Wu JR, Walls JT. Percutaneous balloon aortic valvuloplasty: results in 23 patients. Am J Cardiol 1984;53:194–7.
8. Rossi RI, Manica JL, Petraco R, et al. Balloon aortic valvuloplasty for congenital aortic stenosis using the femoral and the carotid artery approach: a 16-year experience from a single center. Catheter Cardiovasc Interv 2011;78:84–90.
9. Fischer DR, Ettedgui JA, Park SC, et al. Carotid artery approach for balloon dilatation of aortic valve stenosis in the neonate. J Am Coll Cardiol 1990;15:1633–6.
10. Weber HS. Catheter management of aortic valve stenosis in neonates and children. Catheter Cardiovasc Interv 2006;67:947–55.

11. Beekman RH, Rocchini AP, Andes A. Balloon valvuloplasty for critical aortic stenosis in the newborn: influence of new catheter technology. J Am Coll Cardiol 1991;17:1172–6.

12. Dua JS, Osborne NJ, Tometzki AJ, et al. Axillary artery approach for balloon valvoplasty in young infants with severe aortic valve stenosis: medium-term results. Catheter Cardiovasc Interv 2006;68:929–35.

13. Hausdorf G, Schneider M, Schirmer KR, et al. Anterograde balloon valvuloplasty of aortic stenosis in children. Am J Cardiol 1993;71:460–2.

14. Magee AG, Nykanen D, McCrindle BW, et al. Balloon dilation of severe aortic stenosis in the neonate: comparison of anterograde and retrograde catheter approaches. J Am Coll Cardiol 1997;30:1061–6.

15. Mullins CE, Nihill MR, Vick GW, et al. Double balloon technique for dilatation of valvular or vessel stenosis in congenital and acquired heart disease. J Am Coll Cardiol 1987;10:107–14.

16. Beekman RH, Rocchini AP, Crowley DC, et al. Comparison of single and double balloon valvuloplasty in children with aortic stenosis. J Am Coll Cardiol 1988;12:480–5.

17. De Giovanni JV, Edgar RA, Cranston A. Adenosine induced transient cardiac standstill in catheter interventional procedures for congenital heart disease. Heart 1998;80:330–3.

18. Daehnert I, Rotzsch C, Wiener M, et al. Rapid right ventricular pacing is an alternative to adenosine in catheter interventional procedures for congenital heart disease. Heart 2004;90:1047–50.

19. Mehta C, Desai T, Shebani S, et al. J. Rapid ventricular pacing for catheter interventions in congenital aortic stenosis and coarctation: effectiveness, safety, and rate titration for optimal results. J Interv Cardiol 2010;23:7–13.

20. Karagöz T, Aypar E, Erdoğan I, et al. Congenital aortic stenosis: a novel technique for ventricular pacing during valvuloplasty. Catheter Cardiovasc Interv 2008;72:527–30.

21. Feltes TF, Bacha E, Beekman RH 3rd, et al, American Heart Association Congenital Cardiac Defects Committee of the Council on Cardiovascular Disease in the Young, Council on Clinical Cardiology, Council on Cardiovascular Radiology and Intervention. Indications for cardiac catheterization and intervention in pediatric cardiac disease: a scientific statement from the American Heart Association. Circulation 2011;123:2607–52.

22. McElhinney DB, Lock JE, Keane JF, et al. Left heart growth, function, and reintervention after balloon aortic valvuloplasty for neonatal aortic stenosis. Circulation 2005;111:451–8.

23. Waight DJ, Hijazi ZM. Balloon aortic valvuloplasty: the single-wire technique. J Interv Cardiol 2004;17:21–2.

24. Zyblewski SC, Shirali GS, Forbus GA, et al. Initial experience with a miniaturized multiplane transesophageal probe in small infants undergoing cardiac operations. Ann Thorac Surg 2010;89:1990–4.

25. Sholler GF, Keane JF, Perry SB, et al. Balloon dilation of congenital aortic valve stenosis. Results and influence of technical and morphological features on outcome. Circulation 1988;78:351–60.

26. Harris JP, Nanda NC, Moxley R, et al. Myocardial perforation due to temporary transvenous pacing catheters in pediatric patients. Cathet Cardiovasc Diagn 1984;10:329–33.

27. Brown DW, Dipilato AE, Chong EC, et al. Aortic valve reinterventions after balloon aortic valvuloplasty for congenital aortic stenosis intermediate and late follow-up. J Am Coll Cardiol 2010;56:1740–9.

28. Fratz S, Gildein HP, Balling G, et al. Aortic valvuloplasty in pediatric patients substantially postpones the need for aortic valve surgery: a single-center experience of 188 patients after up to 17.5 years of follow-up. Circulation 2008;117:1201–6.

29. McCrindle BW. Independent predictors of immediate results of percutaneous balloon aortic valvotomy in children. Valvuloplasty and Angioplasty of Congenital Anomalies (VACA) Registry Investigators. Am J Cardiol 1996;77:286–93.

30. Balmer C, Beghetti M, Fasnacht M, et al. Balloon aortic valvoplasty in paediatric patients: progressive aortic regurgitation is common. Heart 2004;90:77–81.

31. Burrows PE, Benson LN, Williams WG, et al. Iliofemoral arterial complications of balloon angioplasty for systemic obstructions in infants and children. Circulation 1990;82:1697–704.

32. Vermilion RP, Snider AR, Bengur AR, et al. Doppler evaluation of femoral arteries in children after aortic balloon valvuloplasty or coarctation balloon angioplasty. Pediatr Cardiol 1993;14:13–8.

33. Inoue H, Muneuchi J, Ohno T, et al. Central retinal artery occlusion following transcatheter balloon aortic valvuloplasty in an adolescent with aortic valvular stenosis. Pediatr Cardiol 2008;29:830–3.

34. Carpenter GA, Shapiro SR, Cockerham JT, et al. Cardiac dysrhythmias before and after balloon aortic valvuloplasty in children. Am J Cardiol 1992;70:694–5.

35. Ewert P, Bertram H, Breuer J, et al. Balloon valvuloplasty in the treatment of congenital aortic valve stenosis—a retrospective multicenter survey of more than 1000 patients. Int J Cardiol 2011;149:182–5.

36. McCrindle BW, Blackstone EH, Williams WG, et al. Are outcomes of surgical versus transcatheter balloon valvotomy equivalent in neonatal critical aortic stenosis? Circulation 2001;104:I152–8.

Balloon Aortic Valvuloplasty in the Transcatheter Aortic Valve Replacement Era

Sammy Elmariah, MD, MPH[a,b], Dabit Arzamendi, MD, MSc[a,b],
Igor F. Palacios, MD[a,b],*

KEYWORDS

- Balloon aortic valvuloplasty
- Transcatheter aortic valve replacement
- Calcific aortic stenosis • Heart valve disease

In the United States, heart valve disease is estimated to affect 4.2 to 5.6 million people and to contribute to more than 25,000 deaths annually.[1–3] Calcific aortic valve disease, which frequently culminates in severe aortic valve stenosis (AS), is the most common cause of valvular heart disease in the Western world, present in more than 20% of older adults,[4,5] and leading to $1 billion in US health care expenditures.[6] Moreover, critical AS is prevalent in as much as 2% to 3% of the North American population older than 75 years of age, and its prevalence is rising as the population ages.[7] Surgical aortic valve replacement (SAVR) has historically been the only durable treatment of patients with symptomatic severe AS and asymptomatic patients with severe AS undergoing another cardiac surgery.[8] Although SAVR is routinely performed with relatively low mortality,[9,10] up to one-third of patients are precluded from surgery because of advanced age and comorbid conditions,[11] despite a dismal average survival of only 2 to 3 years in patients with symptomatic severe AS who do not undergo surgery.[8,12]

Percutaneous balloon aortic valvuloplasty (BAV) was first performed in patients with acquired severe AS by Cribier in 1985, at which time it was anticipated to be an alternative to SAVR.[13] In the current era, BAV is recommended for the treatment of severe AS in children and young adults,[8] but initial enthusiasm surrounding this technique as an alternative to SAVR in older patients with calcific AS waned because of the perceived failure of the procedure to alter the natural history of calcific severe AS and because of significant initial procedural morbidity.[14–16] Despite data suggesting that technical and procedural advances have decreased procedural complication rates in high-risk patients,[17–19] prolongation of survival has not been demonstrated.[20–22] Consequently, BAV has been reserved as a palliative procedure for high-risk patients who cannot undergo valve replacement, either surgical or transcatheter, or as a bridge to surgery in hemodynamically unstable patients.[8]

More recently, transcatheter aortic valve replacement (TAVR) has emerged as a viable alternative to SAVR in inoperable patients or in those with high surgical risk.[23,24] Although this advance is considered the end of BAV by some, this viewpoint has been largely refuted by the continued interest and use of the procedure throughout the interventional community, in part because of

a Interventional Cardiology, Cardiology Division, Massachusetts General Hospital, Harvard Medical School, 55 Fruit Street, GBR 800, Boston, MA 02114, USA
b Structural Heart Disease, Cardiology Division, Massachusetts General Hospital, Harvard Medical School, 55 Fruit Street, GBR 800, Boston, MA 02114, USA
* Corresponding author. Interventional Cardiology, 55 Fruit Street, GBR 800, Massachusetts General Hospital, Boston, MA 02114.
E-mail address: ipalacios@partners.org

Intervent Cardiol Clin 1 (2012) 129–137
doi:10.1016/j.iccl.2011.11.001
2211-7458/12/$ – see front matter © 2012 Elsevier Inc. All rights reserved.

TAVR. Here we review the indications, technical aspects, and outcomes of BAV for calcific aortic stenosis as well as discuss the current role of BAV in the TAVR era.

PATIENT SELECTION AND INDICATIONS

Calcific AS is a progressive disease that remains asymptomatic for several decades. With the onset of symptoms, typically dyspnea, angina, heart failure, or syncope,[12] expected survival decreases dramatically with 1-year, 2-year, and 3-year survival rates of 57%, 37%, and 25%, respectively.[25] Once symptoms develop, SAVR should be performed as the standard of care (American College of Cardiology/American Heart Association (ACC/AHA) class I recommendation).[8] The role of BAV should consequently be considered only in those who are not surgical candidates. In these high-risk patients, the ACC/AHA guidelines state that BAV may be considered (class IIb recommendation) as a bridge to surgery in hemodynamically unstable patients or as a palliative option in inoperable candidates.[8] In addition, BAV is widely accepted as beneficial in children and adolescents with bicuspid AS who are symptomatic or who have electrocardiographic changes, either at rest or with exercise, and a peak gradient greater than 50 mm Hg or in asymptomatic patients with a peak gradient greater than 60 mm Hg.[8] In these young patients without heavy valve calcification, BAV often results in significant durable improvements in measures of AS severity.[26–29]

In addition to these accepted guidelines, our institution has found BAV useful in several other clinical situations (**Table 1**). First, we believe that BAV may have a role in patients with rheumatic AS. The lack of heavy leaflet calcification and the presence of commissural fusion may be amenable to balloon commissurotomy, because it is in the mitral position, and recent data support this notion.[30] BAV may also be used to reduce the risk of major noncardiac surgery in patients with severe calcific AS, whether symptomatic or asymptomatic.[31,32] As an extension of the ACC/AHA recommendation for BAV as a bridge to SAVR,[8] we and others have used BAV as a bridge to TAVR.[33] Although TAVR may ultimately be feasible in unstable patients, the current availability of TAVR technologies solely within clinical trials often limits their use in this regard. Such instability also precludes the extensive evaluations necessitated by ongoing TAVR trials. In a subset of patients with left ventricular dysfunction, the

---

Table 1
Indications for BAV

ACC/AHA Guidelines	
Class I	Young patient with symptomatic AS and peak transvalvular gradient ≥50 mm Hg[a]
	Young patient with asymptomatic AS and peak transvalvular gradient ≥60 mm Hg[a]
	Young patient with asymptomatic AS and ST or T wave changes on electrocardiogram at rest or with exercise and a peak transvalvular gradient ≥50 mm Hg[a]
Class IIa	Young patient with asymptomatic AS and peak transvalvular gradient ≥50 mm Hg who desires to play sports or become pregnant[a]
	In a young patient with AS, BAV is probably preferable to SAVR
Class IIb	Bridge to SAVR in an unstable patient with symptomatic calcific AS
	Palliation in an inoperable patient with symptomatic calcific AS
Massachusetts General Hospital Practice	
	Symptomatic AS caused by rheumatic heart disease
	Bridge to TAVR in a patient with symptomatic calcific AS
	Cardiogenic shock in a patient with severe calcific AS
	Patient with symptomatic calcific AS in need of other major surgery
	Diagnostic evaluation of symptoms in a patient with severe calcific AS and another potentially responsible comorbid condition

[a] Refers to peak-to-peak gradient during catheterization.

Data from Bonow RO, Carabello BA, Chatterjee K, et al. 2008 focused update incorporated into the ACC/AHA 2006 guidelines for the management of patients with valvular heart disease: a report of the American College of Cardiology/American Heart Association Task Force on Practice Guidelines (Writing Committee to Revise the 1998 Guidelines for the Management of Patients With Valvular Heart Disease): endorsed by the Society of Cardiovascular Anesthesiologists, Society for Cardiovascular Angiography and Interventions, and Society of Thoracic Surgeons. Circulation 2008;118(15):e523–661.

modest alleviation of the aortic valve obstruction seen with BAV has resulted in significant improvements in left ventricular function. In so doing, BAV before SAVR in high-risk patients has been associated with improved surgical outcomes.[34,35] Similarly, patients precluded from TAVR trials because of severe left ventricular dysfunction may qualify for trials if significant improvements in left ventricular ejection fraction are seen after BAV. We have had success in treating patients with severe aortic stenosis and cardiogenic shock with BAV. In a series of patients from Massachusetts General Hospital, emergent BAV in this setting resulted in an increase in systolic blood pressure from 77 ± 3 to 116 ± 8 mm Hg ($P = .0001$) and in cardiac index from 1.84 ± 0.13 to 2.24 ± 0.15 L/min/m^2 ($P = .06$).[36] In rare situations, we have used BAV as a diagnostic technique to definitively determine whether patient symptoms are secondary to severe AS before subjecting them to more high-risk procedures such as SAVR or TAVR. Such cases have included patients with systolic dysfunction, restrictive and constrictive heart disease, severe lung disease, mixed valve disease, neurologic dysfunction, deconditioned state, and low-gradient, low-output AS.

Given that BAV is mostly used for palliation in patients without other therapeutic options, we consider the only absolute contraindications to be the presence of left ventricular thrombus. In addition, significant obstructive disease within the left main coronary artery confers high procedural mortality. Aortic valvuloplasty has been performed safely in patients with cardiogenic shock, severe aortic regurgitation, and, as described, severe peripheral arterial disease.[36–38] However, when the goal of BAV is to bridge a patient to either SAVR or TAVR, estimation of short-term mortality is of great benefit. Consequently, we evaluated predictors of short-term survival in 292 patients undergoing their first BAV from 2001 to 2007 at the Mount Sinai Hospital.[39] Within this cohort, we found that of all the individual variables within the EuroSCORE and baseline hemodynamic data,[40] critical status (ventricular tachycardia or fibrillation, aborted sudden death, preoperative ventilation, preoperative inotropic support, intra-aortic balloon counterpulsation, or preoperative anuria or oliguria), renal dysfunction (creatinine >2.26 mg/dL), right atrial pressure, and low-cardiac output (≤4.1 L/min) were highly predictive of 30-day mortality after BAV.[39] Using these variables, we derived a clinical prediction score, the CRRAC (critical status, renal dysfunction, right atrial pressure, and cardiac output) the AV risk score (**Fig. 1**), which identified high-risk patients

with better discrimination than either the additive or logistic EuroSCORE. When categorized into tertiles, the increase in risk seemed concentrated among individuals in the highest tertile (score ≥20) of risk score, such that compared with the lowest tertile (score ≤10), the hazard ratio for 30-day mortality was 1.10 (95% confidence interval [CI] 0.34–3.61; $P = .87$) in the middle tertile and 5.82 (95% CI 2.38–14.19; $P<.0001$) in the highest tertile. Similarly, the 30-day survival of individuals in the highest tertile of risk score was 72.2%, in contrast to 94.4% and 92.2% for those in the lowest and middle tertiles, respectively (see **Fig. 1**).[39] Although validation of the CRRAC the AV risk score is yet to be performed, it may identify a high-risk cohort in which bridging BAV is less likely to succeed.

PROCEDURAL DETAILS

Percutaneous BAV can be performed via the retrograde approach, and in rare situations when the iliofemoral vasculature or aorta are prohibitively diseased, the anterograde approach, with similar hemodynamic results.[37] When the extent of peripheral arterial disease is unknown, we perform an iliofemoral angiogram in all patients after achieving insertion of a 5-Fr arterial introducer. For those patients with reduced iliofemoral artery caliber, the anterograde approach should be considered.

The anterograde approach is the more challenging, requiring a higher grade of experience because of the potential damage of the mitral valve. Right femoral venous access is obtained in the usual fashion and transseptal puncture performed using a modified Brockenbrough needle and a Mullins sheath (Medtronic, Inc., Minneapolis, MN, USA) to allow for left atrial entry. A balloon wedge catheter is advanced through the Mullins sheath into the left ventricle and then anterograde through the stenotic aortic valve. The balloon should remain partially inflated during passage from the left atrium to the aorta to minimize the risk of entangling the mitral subvalvular apparatus. A soft 0.97-mm (0.038-inch) exchange wire is advanced through the catheter into the ascending and descending aorta. The wire is snared in the descending aorta with a gooseneck snare and externalized through the femoral artery. An arteriovenous loop is created that allows the valvuloplasty balloon to be advanced through the septum and positioned across the aortic valve. The chosen dilating balloon catheter is then advanced anterograde across the mitral valve, placed across the aortic valve, and valvuloplasty performed during rapid pacing to maintain

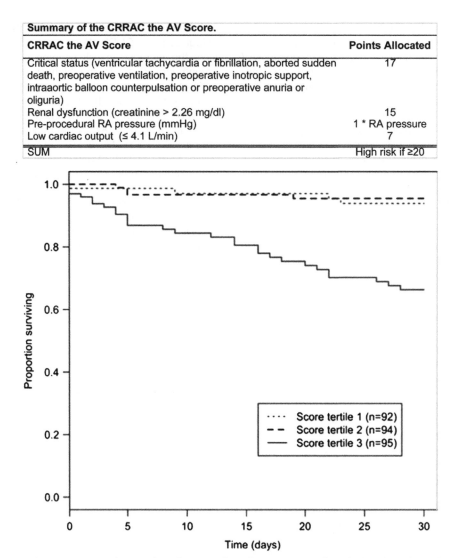

Summary of the CRRAC the AV Score.	
CRRAC the AV Score	**Points Allocated**
Critical status (ventricular tachycardia or fibrillation, aborted sudden death, preoperative ventilation, preoperative inotropic support, intraaortic balloon counterpulsation or preoperative anuria or oliguria)	17
Renal dysfunction (creatinine > 2.26 mg/dl)	15
Pre-procedural RA pressure (mmHg)	1 * RA pressure
Low cardiac output (≤ 4.1 L/min)	7
SUM	High risk if ≥20

Fig. 1. CRRAC the AV score. Predictors of 30-day mortality after BAV were identified and a risk prediction model constructed based on critical status, renal dysfunction, pre-BAV right atrial pressure, and cardiac output. As shown in Kaplan-Meier curves stratified by tertile of the CRRAC the AV score, patients within the highest tertile (score ≥20) had poor survival. (*From* Elmariah S, Lubitz SA, Shah AM, et al. A novel clinical prediction rule for 30-day mortality following balloon aortic valuloplasty: the CRRAC the AV score. Catheter Cardiovasc Interv 2011;78(1):116; with permission.)

balloon stability. Care is taken to maintain the wire/catheter loop within the left ventricle to avoid injury to the mitral valve. After 2 or 3 inflations, the balloon is removed, keeping the arteriovenous loop in place. The Mullins sheath is then advanced to the left ventricle to reassess the transvalvular gradient (**Fig. 2**).

In performing BAV via the retrograde approach, the common femoral artery is cannulated as mentioned earlier and iliofemoral angiography performed. If the puncture site is adequate and there is no significant stenosis of the common femoral, preclosure using 2 Perclose ProGlide (Abbott Vascular, Santa Clara, CA, USA) suture systems can be performed. The devices should be rotated such that the second device is deployed 90° from the first. The 10-Fr to 14-Fr sheath is then inserted over the wire depending on the valvuloplasty balloon size to be used. Preclosure of the vascular access site results in immediate hemostasis on completion of the procedure and has greatly reduced the vascular complications associated with BAV.[18] We most frequently cross the stenotic valve using a 6-Fr Amplatz left catheter and a straight 0.89-mm (0.035-inch) guidewire. We prefer the Judkins right or a multipurpose catheter

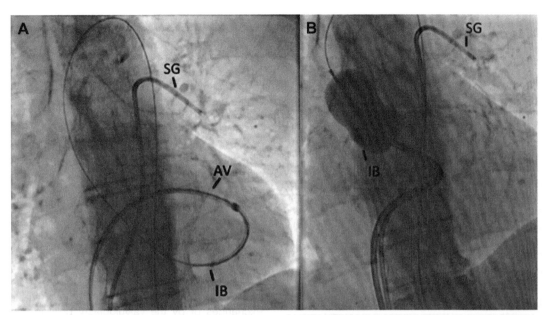

Fig. 2. Anterograde BAV. Fluoroscopic images showing the stages of anterograde BAV. (*A*) A Mullins sheath is advanced via transseptal puncture into the left ventricle. A wire is then advanced into the descending aorta and snared from the femoral artery. To avoid injury to the mitral valve, a large arteriovenous (AV) loop is created within the left ventricle. An Inoue balloon catheter (IB) is then advanced while partially inflated through the left ventricle and across the aortic valve. (*B*) BAV is performed while pulling the Inoue balloon (IB) catheter against the aortic valve. SG, Swan-Ganz catheter.

if the aortic root is more horizontal. The straight anteroposterior projection or slight left cranial angulation helps to identify the right and left cusps. The Amplatz catheter is then exchanged for a double-lumen pigtail catheter over an extra-stiff wire, the distal end of which should be manually curved to increase the wire and to decrease the risks of ventricular perforation during the valvuloplasty. After hemodynamic measurements are obtained, the pigtail catheter is exchanged for the valvuloplasty balloon. We select the initial balloon size to approximate the left ventricular outflow dimension. The valvuloplasty balloon is fully inflated during rapid ventricular pacing at a rate of 180 beats per minute once the systolic blood pressure is reduced by at least half. Valvuloplasty can be performed without rapid pacing, although this has been shown to improve balloon stability.[41] After 2 or 3 balloon inflations, the valvuloplasty balloon is removed, keeping the wire inside the left ventricle, and the double-lumen pigtail catheter is reinserted to assess the effectiveness of the valvuloplasty (**Fig. 3**). If a suboptimal result is obtained, the valvuloplasty can be repeated

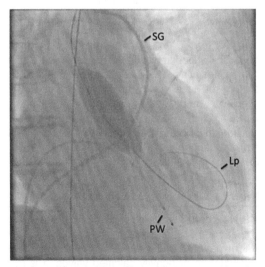

Fig. 3. Retrograde BAV. Fluoroscopic images showing the stages of retrograde BAV. The stenotic aortic valve is crossed with a straight wire using an Amplatz left catheter. After exchanging for a stiff wire with generous distal loop (Lp), the chosen balloon catheter is advanced across the valve and inflated during rapid ventricular pacing. PW, temporary pacing wire; SG, Swan-Ganz catheter.

using a larger balloon. At the completion of the procedure, closure of the arteriotomy is performed using the preclosure device sutures.

PROCEDURAL COMPLICATIONS
Death

In-hospital mortality occurs in 5% to 8% of patients, with 1 to 2% expiring within the catheterization laboratory.[24,42–44] Most of these deaths occur either as the result of fatal complications of the procedure, such as arrhythmia, aortic rupture, or ventricular perforation, or because of a progressive heart failure and cardiogenic shock in patients with severely depressed left ventricular function. In our experience, significant stenosis of the left main coronary artery is a significant predictor of procedural mortality.

Vascular Complication

Given that vascular access for BAV is performed on frail patients of advanced age, most of whom have significant peripheral arterial disease, vascular access complications are among the most common. Vascular complications, including perforation, dissection, hematoma, pseudoaneurysm, or arterial-venous fistula formation, retroperitoneal bleeding, or atheroembolization occurred in as many as 25% of patients in early studies.[14,15,36] Moreover, these major vascular complications are associated with increased mortality and morbidity; therefore adequate arterial access in these patients is essential. Peripheral angioplasty balloons from 7 to 10 mm should be on hand because if vascular perforation occurs rapid action can be lifesaving. The introduction of the vascular closure devices has dramatically reduced the need for surgery and blood transfusion.[18,45] Vascular closure devices, perhaps the most significant advance in BAV over the last 25 years, have reduced the rate of vascular complications[44] to approximately 5%.[18,43,45]

Severe Aortic Valve Regurgitation

Massive aortic regurgitation after BAV can be a fatal complication that occurs in approximately 1% of patients during BAV.[42,43] In patients with small stature or heavily calcified valves, it is recommended to dilate the valve in a stepwise fashion from the small-sized to the larger-sized balloon. If massive regurgitation occurs and the patient is hemodynamically stable, urgent surgery or TAVR has to be considered. In stable patients, the valve replacement procedure can be postponed and performed electively.

Stroke

The occurrence of clinically apparent cerebral events is less than 2%.[24,42,43] These events are believed to be caused by embolism of atherosclerotic debris from the ascending aorta or the valve cusps during attempts to cross the valve or during balloon inflation. Thrombus formation on catheters or wires within the ascending aorta and left ventricle is also possible. Patients should consequently be treated with 50 to 70 units/kg of heparin at the beginning of the procedure. Aggressive crossing of the valve should be avoided, and the wire and the catheter should be retrieved and flushed every 3 minutes if the valve is difficult to cross.

Left Ventricular Perforation and Tamponade

Cardiac perforation and tamponade during BAV can be caused by the stiff wire used for catheter exchanges or by the valvuloplasty balloon itself in approximately 1% of cases.[43,45] Tamponade is most often a result of sudden ventricular movement of the balloon during inflation, although positioning of the balloon more ventricular than aortic can also contribute. To avoid left ventricular perforation, it is imperative to create a large curve on the distal tip of the stiff wire. This strategy helps to maintain balloon stability during inflations and also helps to prevent wire perforation. In addition, by reducing cardiac output, rapid ventricular pacing helps to reduce sudden movement of the valvuloplasty balloon.

Electrophysiologic Complications

Atrioventricular heart block may occur with BAV as a consequence of direct trauma to the conduction system. Atrioventricular block is more commonly seen in those with underlying conduction system disease such as preexisting bundle branch block and in those with small left ventricular outflow tracts. In our experience, atrioventricular block can be transient, although pacemaker implantation has been reported in 1.5% of patients after BAV.[46]

Ventricular arrhythmias are frequent during the wire and balloon manipulation inside the left ventricle. Simple repositioning of the wire or releasing tension may be enough to end these arrhythmias. On rare occasions, sustained ventricular tachycardia or fibrillation can occur, necessitating resuscitation and cardioversion.[43]

PATIENT OUTCOMES

According to early data from 2 large registries as well as from our institution, the Massachusetts

General Hospital, BAV resulted in significant acute improvement in aortic valve area (average of 0.3 cm^2), mean aortic valve gradients, cardiac output, symptoms, and functional class; however, the procedure was associated with significant periprocedural and short-term morbidity and mortality.[14,15,36] In the National Heart, Lung and Blood Institute Balloon Valvuloplasty registry, almost one-third of 674 high-risk elderly patients experienced a significant complication such as vascular injury, embolic event, or myocardial infarction. Furthermore, long-term survival after BAV was poor with 1-year, 2-year, and 3-year survival rates of 55%, 35% and 23%, respectively,[16] rates almost identical to the survival seen in patients with untreated severe AS.[25] Early hemodynamic improvements obtained immediately after BAV also abated with accelerated valve recoil and restenosis after the procedure.[47]

Recent studies have maintained the lack of survival benefit after BAV compared with historical survival rates with medical therapy alone,[24] although there may be a slight improvement in survival with repeated BAV.[42] Symptomatic relief can be expected to last 6 to 12 months,[16] although 1 recent report documented improvement for as long as 18 months.[42] Within the PARTNER (Placement of Aortic Transcatheter Valve) trial, the mortality rate for patients within the standard therapy arm, 85% of whom underwent BAV, was 50% at 1 year,[24] a rate consistent with previous findings.[16]

IMPLICATIONS OF TAVR FOR BAV

Some have considered advances in SAVR techniques and the advent of TAVR to be the death of BAV. However, the procedural volume for BAV has increased exponentially since the introduction of TAVR 5 years ago.[43,45] The prolonged clinical evaluation often necessary for inclusion in TAVR trials frequently necessitates BAV as a bridging procedure. In addition, strict inclusion and exclusion criteria for TAVR clinical trials have driven a significant number of patients to seek BAV or high-risk SAVR instead. These factors may change once TAVR is approved for use outside clinical trials. However, BAV is a component of the TAVR procedure, necessitating interventional cardiologists to maintain the skills involved in performing BAV. Conversely, because TAVR is more widely adopted, previous familiarity with BAV facilitates interventionalists' comfort with TAVR. For now, BAV and TAVR are intimately intertwined. The forthcoming ubiquitous implementation of TAVR is sure to continue driving the resurgence of BAV.

FUTURE DIRECTIONS

Antiproliferative drugs, such as rapamycin and paclitaxel, have revolutionized interventional cardiology as a treatment of restenosis after coronary stenting. These agents act via inhibition of vascular smooth muscle cell proliferation and migration, steps critical for stent restenosis.[48,49] Assumptions that these agents may similarly inhibit valve myofibroblasts has led to the hypothesis that antiproliferative agents may slow aortic valve restenosis after BAV. A recent study evaluated the potential for local delivery of paclitaxel to the aortic valve using a paclitaxel-eluting valvuloplasty balloon in pigs and found that drug concentrations within the valve were at therapeutic levels.[50] Adopting a similar rationale, external beam radiation therapy (EBRT) has been used in an attempt to slow valve restenosis. Within a small pilot study, 21% of patients receiving EBRT after BAV developed restenosis at 1 year compared with the historically expected rate of ~80%.[51] These preliminary results are intriguing, but further study is needed to evaluate the use of antiproliferative agents and radiation therapy in managing calcific aortic valve disease.

REFERENCES

1. Thom T, Haase N, Rosamond W, et al. Heart disease and stroke statistics–2006 update: a report from the American Heart Association Statistics Committee and Stroke Statistics Subcommittee. Circulation 2006;113(6):e85–151.
2. Elmariah S, Mohler ER 3rd. The pathogenesis and treatment of the valvulopathy of aortic stenosis: beyond the SEAS. Curr Cardiol Rep 2010;12(2): 125–32.
3. Goldbarg SH, Elmariah S, Miller MA, et al. Insights into degenerative aortic valve disease. J Am Coll Cardiol 2007;50(13):1205–13.
4. Stewart BF, Siscovick D, Lind BK, et al. Clinical factors associated with calcific aortic valve disease. Cardiovascular Health Study. J Am Coll Cardiol 1997;29(3):630–4.
5. Stritzke J, Linsel-Nitschke P, Markus MR, et al. Association between degenerative aortic valve disease and long-term exposure to cardiovascular risk factors: results of the longitudinal population-based KORA/MONICA survey. Eur Heart J 2009;30(16): 2044–53.
6. Moura LM, Ramos SF, Zamorano JL, et al. Rosuvastatin affecting aortic valve endothelium to slow the progression of aortic stenosis. J Am Coll Cardiol 2007;49(5):554–61.
7. Lindroos M, Kupari M, Heikkila J, et al. Prevalence of aortic valve abnormalities in the elderly: an

echocardiographic study of a random population sample. J Am Coll Cardiol 1993;21(5):1220–5.

8. Bonow RO, Carabello BA, Chatterjee K, et al. 2008 focused update incorporated into the ACC/AHA 2006 guidelines for the management of patients with valvular heart disease: a report of the American College of Cardiology/American Heart Association Task Force on Practice Guidelines (Writing Committee to Revise the 1998 Guidelines for the Management of Patients With Valvular Heart Disease): endorsed by the Society of Cardiovascular Anesthesiologists, Society for Cardiovascular Angiography and Interventions, and Society of Thoracic Surgeons. Circulation 2008;118(15):e523–661.

9. Astor BC, Kaczmarek RG, Hefflin B, et al. Mortality after aortic valve replacement: results from a nationally representative database. Ann Thorac Surg 2000;70(6):1939–45.

10. Rankin JS, Hammill BG, Ferguson TB Jr, et al. Determinants of operative mortality in valvular heart surgery. J Thorac Cardiovasc Surg 2006;131(3):547–57.

11. Iung B, Cachier A, Baron G, et al. Decision-making in elderly patients with severe aortic stenosis: why are so many denied surgery? Eur Heart J 2005; 26(24):2714–20.

12. Ross J Jr, Braunwald E. Aortic stenosis. Circulation 1968;38(Suppl 1):61–7.

13. Cribier A, Savin T, Saoudi N, et al. Percutaneous transluminal valvuloplasty of acquired aortic stenosis in elderly patients: an alternative to valve replacement? Lancet 1986;1(8472):63–7.

14. McKay RG. The Mansfield Scientific Aortic Valvuloplasty Registry: overview of acute hemodynamic results and procedural complications. J Am Coll Cardiol 1991;17(2):485–91.

15. Percutaneous balloon aortic valvuloplasty. Acute and 30-day follow-up results in 674 patients from the NHLBI Balloon Valvuloplasty Registry. Circulation 1991;84(6):2383–97.

16. Otto CM, Mickel MC, Kennedy JW, et al. Three-year outcome after balloon aortic valvuloplasty. Insights into prognosis of valvular aortic stenosis. Circulation 1994;89(2):642–50.

17. Sack S, Kahlert P, Khandanpour S, et al. Revival of an old method with new techniques: balloon aortic valvuloplasty of the calcified aortic stenosis in the elderly. Clin Res Cardiol 2008;97(5):288–97.

18. Ben-Dor I, Looser P, Bernardo N, et al. Comparison of closure strategies after balloon aortic valvuloplasty: suture mediated versus collagen based versus manual. Catheter Cardiovasc Interv 2011; 78(1):119–24.

19. Hara H, Pedersen WR, Ladich E, et al. Percutaneous balloon aortic valvuloplasty revisited: time for a renaissance? Circulation 2007;115(12):e334–8.

20. Pedersen WR, Klaassen PJ, Boisjolie CR, et al. Feasibility of transcatheter intervention for severe aortic stenosis in patients > or = 90 years of age: aortic valvuloplasty revisited. Catheter Cardiovasc Interv 2007;70(1):149–54.

21. Shareghi S, Rasouli L, Shavelle DM, et al. Current results of balloon aortic valvuloplasty in high-risk patients. J Invasive Cardiol 2007;19(1):1–5.

22. Lieberman EB, Bashore TM, Hermiller JB, et al. Balloon aortic valvuloplasty in adults: failure of procedure to improve long-term survival. J Am Coll Cardiol 1995;26(6):1522–8.

23. Smith CR, Leon MB, Mack MJ, et al. Transcatheter versus surgical aortic-valve replacement in high-risk patients. N Engl J Med 2011;364(23): 2187–98.

24. Leon MB, Smith CR, Mack M, et al. Transcatheter aortic-valve implantation for aortic stenosis in patients who cannot undergo surgery. N Engl J Med 2010;363(17):1597–607.

25. O'Keefe JH Jr, Vlietstra RE, Bailey KR, et al. Natural history of candidates for balloon aortic valvuloplasty. Mayo Clin Proc 1987;62(11):986–91.

26. Huhta JC, Carpenter RJ Jr, Moise KJ Jr, et al. Prenatal diagnosis and postnatal management of critical aortic stenosis. Circulation 1987;75(3):573–6.

27. Pass RH, Hellenbrand WE. Catheter intervention for critical aortic stenosis in the neonate. Catheter Cardiovasc Interv 2002;55(1):88–92.

28. Rao PS, Jureidini SB. Transumbilical venous, antegrade, snare-assisted balloon aortic valvuloplasty in a neonate with critical aortic stenosis. Cathet Cardiovasc Diagn 1998;45(2):144–8.

29. Beekman RH, Rocchini AP, Andes A. Balloon valvuloplasty for critical aortic stenosis in the newborn: influence of new catheter technology. J Am Coll Cardiol 1991;17(5):1172–6.

30. Rifaie O, El-Itriby A, Zaki T, et al. Immediate and long-term outcome of multiple percutaneous interventions in patients with rheumatic valvular stenosis. EuroIntervention 2010;6(2):227–32.

31. Roth RB, Palacios IF, Block PC. Percutaneous aortic balloon valvuloplasty: its role in the management of patients with aortic stenosis requiring major noncardiac surgery. J Am Coll Cardiol 1989;13(5): 1039–41.

32. Torsher LC, Shub C, Rettke SR, et al. Risk of patients with severe aortic stenosis undergoing noncardiac surgery. Am J Cardiol 1998;81(4):448–52.

33. Tissot CM, Attias D, Himbert D, et al. Reappraisal of percutaneous aortic balloon valvuloplasty as a preliminary treatment strategy in the transcatheter aortic valve implantation era. EuroIntervention 2011; 7(1):49–56.

34. Safian RD, Warren SE, Berman AD, et al. Improvement in symptoms and left ventricular performance after balloon aortic valvuloplasty in patients with aortic stenosis and depressed left ventricular ejection fraction. Circulation 1988;78(5 Pt 1):1181–91.

35. Doguet F, Godin M, Lebreton G, et al. Aortic valve replacement after percutaneous valvuloplasty–an approach in otherwise inoperable patients. Eur J Cardiothorac Surg 2010;38(4):394–9.

36. Moreno PR, Jang IK, Newell JB, et al. The role of percutaneous aortic balloon valvuloplasty in patients with cardiogenic shock and critical aortic stenosis. J Am Coll Cardiol 1994;23(5):1071–5.

37. Block PC, Palacios IF. Comparison of hemodynamic results of anterograde versus retrograde percutaneous balloon aortic valvuloplasty. Am J Cardiol 1987;60(8):659–62.

38. Saia F, Marrozzini C, Ciuca C, et al. Is balloon aortic valvuloplasty safe in patients with significant aortic valve regurgitation? Catheter Cardiovasc Interv 2011. DOI:10.1002/ccd.23092. [Epub ahead of print].

39. Elmariah S, Lubitz SA, Shah AM, et al. A novel clinical prediction rule for 30-day mortality following balloon aortic valuloplasty: the CRRAC the AV score. Catheter Cardiovasc Interv 2011;78(1):112–8.

40. Noshed SA, Roques F, Michel P, et al. European system for cardiac operative risk evaluation (EuroSCORE). Eur J Cardiothorac Surg 1999;16(1):9–13.

41. Witzke C, Don CW, Cubeddu RJ, et al. Impact of rapid ventricular pacing during percutaneous balloon aortic valvuloplasty in patients with critical aortic stenosis: should we be using it? Catheter Cardiovasc Interv 2010;75(3):444–52.

42. Agarwal A, Kini AS, Attanti S, et al. Results of repeat balloon valvuloplasty for treatment of aortic stenosis in patients aged 59 to 104 years. Am J Cardiol 2005; 95(1):43–7.

43. Ben-Dor I, Pichard AD, Satler LF, et al. Complications and outcome of balloon aortic valvuloplasty in high-risk or inoperable patients. JACC Cardiovasc Interv 2010;3(11):1150–6.

44. Don CW, Witzke C, Cubeddu RJ, et al. Comparison of procedural and in-hospital outcomes of percutaneous balloon aortic valvuloplasty in patients >80 years versus patients < or = 80 years. Am J Cardiol 2010;105(12):1815–20.

45. Solomon LW, Fusman B, Jolly N, et al. Percutaneous suture closure for management of large French size arterial puncture in aortic valvuloplasty. J Invasive Cardiol 2001;13(8):592–6.

46. Laynez A, Ben-Dor I, Hauville C, et al. Frequency of cardiac conduction disturbances after balloon aortic valvuloplasty. Am J Cardiol 2011;108(9):1311–5.

47. Bernard Y, Bassand JP, Anguenot T, et al. Aortic valve area evolution after percutaneous aortic valvuloplasty. A prospective trial using a combined Doppler echocardiographic and haemodynamic method. Eur Heart J 1990;11(2):98–107.

48. Poon M, Badimon JJ, Fuster V. Overcoming restenosis with sirolimus: from alphabet soup to clinical reality. Lancet 2002;359(9306):619–22.

49. Wessely R, Schomig A, Kastrati A. Sirolimus and Paclitaxel on polymer-based drug-eluting stents: similar but different. J Am Coll Cardiol 2006;47(4):708–14.

50. Spargias K, Milewski K, Debinski M, et al. Drug delivery at the aortic valve tissues of healthy domestic pigs with a Paclitaxel-eluting valvuloplasty balloon. J Interv Cardiol 2009;22(3):291–8.

51. Pedersen WR, Van Tassel RA, Pierce TA, et al. Radiation following percutaneous balloon aortic valvuloplasty to prevent restenosis (RADAR pilot trial). Catheter Cardiovasc Interv 2006;68(2):183–92.

Looking to the Future of Percutaneous Treatment of Patients with Valvular Heart Disease

Rajeev L. Narayan, MD[a],*, Samin K. Sharma, MD[b]

KEYWORDS

- Percutaneous valve replacement • TAVI
- Percutaneous valve repair • MitraClip • CoreValve
- Edwards SAPIEN valve

The past decade has seen the development of one of the most innovative and novel technologies in interventional cardiology since the development of the coronary stent: the transcatheter replacement and repair of cardiac valves. Before the development of percutaneous valvular technology, interventionalists were limited to the use of balloon valvuloplasty in managing stenotic valves.[1–7] Although this technology had seen success in managing congenital disease, the more complex management of senile calcific and degenerative aortic stenosis was marred by the oft-feared recurrence of stenosis after balloon aortic valvuloplasty (BAV).[2,4] In addition, the percutaneous management of regurgitant lesions evolved even less favorably, and historically these lesions remained within the surgical domain.[8]

As a result of these limitations, and because of the need for percutaneous therapies for patients who cannot undergo open surgical repair or replacement, interventional cardiologists and surgeons have developed a series of endovascular tools specifically aimed at treating valvular disease. Soon, the armamentarium of the structural interventionalist will include not only balloon valvuloplasty but also balloon and self-expanding valve stents,[9] transseptal repair delivery systems,[8] specialized intracardiac and extracardiac imaging for valvular intervention guidance[10] and a host of other technologies that still remain in development. The future of this all-important technology seems bright. On balance, the success of these potent resources depends on the coordinated efforts between large cardiac teams, which include not just the interventionalist but also the noninvasive cardiologist, imaging cardiologist, cardiac surgeon, and numerous other roles that are yet to be determined. This is an exciting era in interventional cardiology, and the emergence of these technologies will likely have vast influence and impact on clinical practice. In this article the current status of these percutaneous technologies is discussed as they pertain to the 2 valves with the greatest overall human experience: the aortic valve and the mitral valve. The projected future expectations of the role of transcatheter intervention in managing complex structural heart disease in the adult are also discussed.

The authors have nothing to disclose in relationship to this article.

[a] Cardiovascular Diseases, Mount Sinai School of Medicine, One Gustave L. Levy Place, New York, NY 10029, USA

[b] Cardiac Catheterization Laboratory, Mount Sinai Heart, Mount Sinai Hospital, One Gustave L. Levy Place, New York, NY 10029, USA

* Corresponding author.

E-mail address: Rajeev.Narayan@mountsinai.org

PERCUTANEOUS MANAGEMENT OF AORTIC VALVE DISEASE
Background

Aortic stenosis is one of the most prevalent valvular heart diseases worldwide, with an estimated 5% of adults older than 75 years living with the condition.[11] It is further predicted that as the population continues to age, there will be an increasing incidence in the diagnosis of senile degenerative aortic stenosis. The condition is devastating, with randomized trial data reporting a 50.7% 1-year mortality after symptom development in conservatively managed patients.[12] Surgical replacement of the aortic valve reduces symptoms and improves survival in patients with aortic stenosis.[13,14] In addition, when performed in patients with few comorbid conditions, surgical aortic valve replacement (SAVR) is associated with a low operative mortality and excellent postoperative outcomes.[15] However, despite the excellent results of SAVR, up to 50% of patients are not given this curative treatment option because of age, high-risk comorbid conditions such as left ventricular dysfunction, and patient preference.[16,17]

The need for less invasive therapies to treat high-risk patients with aortic stenosis resulted in the development of BAV. The first BAV was performed in 1985, and held initial promise as a viable alternative therapy to SAVR for acquired aortic stenosis in elderly patients.[18] However, initial excitement became rapidly tempered after long-term follow-up data revealed the rampant recurrence of restenosis.[19] Although novel approaches, such as external beam radiation after BAV[20] and cutting BAV have been attempted to temper restenosis, long-term benefits have not yet been achieved. The role of BAV in the treatment of aortic stenosis is mainly palliative, or in some patients, used as a bridge to SAVR.[11]

The principle of BAV set the stage for one of the greatest advances in interventional cardiology: the novel approach to aortic valve replacement via a percutaneous approach. Transcatheter aortic valve implantation (TAVI) has evolved in the last decade and has already revolutionized the method of managing aortic valve stenosis in patients who are too ill to safely undergo surgery.[9,12] Since the first TAVI implantation in 2002, more than 20,000 patients worldwide have been treated, with an overall procedural success rate of more than 90% according to the SOURCE (SAPIEN Aortic Bioprosthesis European Outcome) registry.[21] In addition, randomized controlled data are now available from the Placement of Aortic Transcatheter Valves (PARTNER) trial, showing the procedural success as well as the mortality benefit of

TAVI over conservative therapy in extreme-risk patients too sick to undergo surgery, and noninferiority when compared with surgery in high-risk surgical patients.[9,12] Thus this technology is evolving as a potential viable alternative therapeutic option in patients with aortic stenosis.

Current Status

There are at least 14 different percutaneous aortic valves in varying stages of development for clinical use in humans (**Table 1**). Most of these valve technologies are in preclinical development, with a handful undergoing first-in-human placement. The 2 valve systems closest to commercial availability with the greatest data are the Edwards SAPIEN Heart Valve System (Edwards Lifesciences, Irvine, CA, USA) and the CoreValve system (Medtronic, Minneapolis, MN, USA). The Edwards SAPIEN valve is the only valve system that has undergone rigorous testing in a randomized controlled trial (the Placement of Aortic Transcather Valves [PARTNER] trial),[9,12] with a second-generation iteration consisting of a lower profile delivery system and modified valve stent planned for evaluation in the upcoming PARTNER II trial (http://clinicaltrials.gov identifier: NCT01314313). At present, the Edwards SAPIEN valve holds CE Mark approval in Europe and Canada, and is the only system approved by the US Food and Drug Administration (FDA) for clinical implantation. The Medtronic CoreValve system (**Fig. 1**) holds CE Mark approval for clinical use in Europe and Canada, and has extensive registry data showing its safety and efficacy. It is currently undergoing evaluation in a randomized clinical study, the CoreValve US Pivotal Trial (http://clinicaltrials.gov identifier: NCT01240902). Patient enrollment for this trial is already under way, with completion planned for 2012, and presentation of 1-year follow-up data in 2013.

Future Directions for Transcatheter Aortic Valve Technology

Whereas the SAPIEN valve and CoreValve have paved the road toward a novel approach in percutaneously treating aortic valve disease, second-generation valve technologies have burgeoned, and are attempting to overcome some of the shortcomings of first-generation valve technologies.

The Paniagua Heart Valve (Endoluminal Technology Research, Miami, FL, USA) was first implanted in 2005 as compassionate use in a severely ill patient with severe aortic stenosis and severe left ventricle dysfunction.[22] It is

Table 1
Percutaneous aortic valve technologies in development for use in humans

Valve Name	Developing Company	Frame Type	Valve Material	Access Site Size (F)	Delivery Mechanism	Current State of Data	Routes of Delivery	Valve Sizes (mm)
Edwards SAPIEN THV	Edwards Lifesciences	Stainless steel	Bovine pericardium	24–26	Balloon expandable	RCT data available	TA/TF	23, 26
Edwards SAPIEN XT	Edwards Lifesciences	Cobalt chromium	Bovine pericardium	18	Balloon expandable	To be studied in planned RCT	TA/TF	23, 26, 29
CoreValve	Medtronic	Nitinol	Porcine pericardium	18	Self-expandable	To be studied in currently enrolling RCT	TF/SC	26, 29
Paniagua	Endoluminal Technology Research	Cheatham-Platinum	Pericardium	11, 16	Balloon and self-expandable	FIH[22]	TF	20
ATS 3f Entrata	Medtronic	Nitinol	Equine pericardium	NA	NA	NA	TA/TF	NA
AortTx	Hansen Medical	Nitinol	Pericardium	24	Self-expandable	FIH[23]	TF	NA
Direct Flow	Direct Flow Medical	Water-soluble epoxy with radiopaque tracer	Bovine pericardium	18	Balloon expandable with polymer injection to maintain form	FIH[25] RCT planned	TF	23
Lotus	Sadra Medical	Nitinol	Bovine pericardium	21	Self-expandable	FIH	TF	21
Perceval	Sorin Group	Nitinol	Bovine pericardium	NA	Self-expandable	NA	NA	NA
JenaValve	Jenavalve Technology	Nitinol paperclip design	Porcine pericardium	NA	Self-expandable	FIH	TA/TF	NA
Heart Leaflet	Heart Leaflet Technologies	Nitinol	Bovine pericardium	16	Self-expandable	NA	TF	NA
Zegdi	St Jude Medical	Nitinol	Porcine pericardium	24	Self-expandable	NA	NA	25
VXI Heart Valve	ValveXchange	Nitinol	Pericardium	NA	Self-expandable	NA	NA	NA
Lutter	NA	Nitinol	Tissue engineered	NA	Self-expandable	NA	NA	NA
PercValve	ABS	Nanosynthesized ε-nitinol	Nanosynthesized ε-nitinol	10	Self-expandable	NA	NA	NA

Abbreviations: FIH, first-in-human; NA, data currently not available; RCT, randomized controlled trial; SC, subclavian; TA, transapical; TF, transfemoral.
Adapted from Cubeddu RJ, Palacios IF. Percutaneous heart valve replacement and repair: advances and future potential. Expert Rev Cardiovasc Ther 2009;7(7):811–21.

A

B

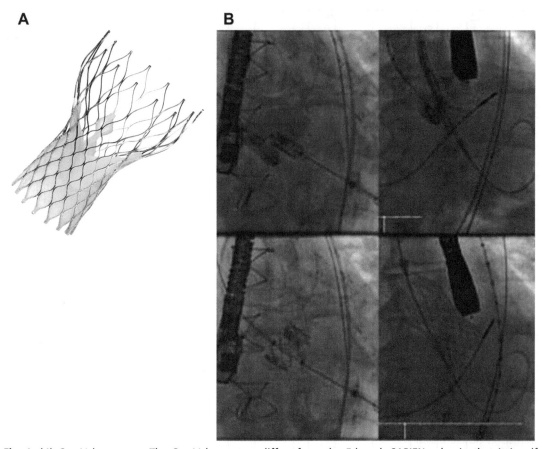

Fig. 1. (*A*) CoreValve system. The CoreValve system differs from the Edwards SAPIEN valve in that it is self-expanding and made from nitinol. It is composed of a porcine pericardial valve mounted on this valve stent frame. The design has 3 distinct levels with varying radial and hoop strength. The CoreValve system is an investigational device and is limited by US law to investigational use. CoreValve is a registered trademark of Medtronic CV Luxembourg S.A.R.L. (*B*) Fluoroscopic deployment of the CoreValve system. The valve is positioned and partially deployed in the left ventricular outflow tract. At this stage, the valve can be retrieved and repositioned. After confirmation of location, the valve can be fully deployed. At final placement, the valve is positioned from the left ventricular outflow tract extending into the aorta. (*From* Cheung A, Soon JL. Transcatheter aortic valve replacement: where will we be in 5 years? Curr Opin Cardiol 2011;26:107; with permission; and *Courtesy of* Medtronic, Minneapolis, MN.)

a biologic valve with a 2-mm collapsed profile, manually crimped on a delivery balloon. It can be implanted via an 11-F or 16-F sheath, depending on the mounting frame and the final valve diameter. Althoughacute hemodynamic results were impressive, the patient died on day 5 after the procedure, with normal valve function on echocardiography before death.

The Lotus Valve (Sadra Medical, Saratoga, CA, USA) is a self-expanding valve system available in a 23-mm size for clinical evaluation. Its unique characteristic is its ability for in vivo performance assessment and repositioning before final deployment. The system includes a 21-F delivery catheter with the valve made of bovine pericardial leaflets attached to a nitinol stent frame. An external sealing membrane fills the gaps between the prosthesis and the native aortic annulus. The system is shaped in 2 distinct formats: (1) a longitudinal form, with a small profile, used for entrance through the sheath and around the aortic arch and (2) a postvalve crossing form, at which time the outer catheter is pulled back, allowing for radial expansion and loss of height, changing the overall shape. The valve can then be repositioned and manipulated until final position is obtained, and is then released. During the entire process of positioning, cardiac flow is preserved, and rapid ventricular pacing becomes unnecessary. The Lotus Valve has been implanted in a 93-year-old patient using a 21-F sheath with excellent hemodynamic results at 90 days.[23]

The Direct Flow Medical valve (Direct Flow Medical, Santa Rosa, CA, USA) is a repositionable valve consisting of 2 inflatable rings linked by a Dacron fabric cuff attached to bovine pericardial leaflets. These rings are provisionally inflated and fixed in position with contrast and saline, during which time repositioning can take place as necessary. Once in final position, the solution is exchanged for a biocompatible solidifying inflation medium that forms the final support structure. This valve is available in 23-mm, 25-mm and 27-mm sizes and has been temporarily tested in the operating room before planned SAVR. Seven successful implants with good hemodynamic results were achieved without significant aortic insufficiency and only 1 procedural failure.[23,24] Further testing took place in a series of 15 patients with severe aortic stenosis who were at high surgical risk for SAVR. In this series, successful implantation occurred in 12 patients, with 11 patients discharged with a permanent implant. Of those patients, 1 patient developed a stroke, and 1 patient died. The 10 surviving patients with permanent implants were followed, and echocardiographic imaging showed significant hemodynamic improvement and increase in aortic valve area at 30 day follow-up.[25]

Numerous other valves, with characteristics further outlined in **Table 1**, are in development for use in humans and are at varying stages of development. The AorTx device (Hansen Medical, Mountain View, CA) consists of a pericardial tissue valve attached to a self-expanding nitinol frame that unrolls to a solid cylindrical shape to anchor in the annulus. The design allows the valve to be folded rather than compressed before deployment. The JenaValve system (JenaValve Technology, GmbH, Munich, Germany) includes 3 basic components: the porcine valve, the JenaClip nitinol stent frame, and the delivery catheter. Its main advantage is its ability to be completely repositionable and retrievable. The Perceval Valve (Sorin Group, Milan, Italy) is a self-expandable bovine pericardial valve based on the surgical Perceval S prosthesis. The frame is made of nitinol and designed to adapt to the anatomy of the aortic root and the sinuses of Valsalva, with 3 additional posts that reinforce fixation to the native valve. The design is meant to minimize the occurrence of paravalvular leak after implantation. The PercValve (Advanced Bioprosthesis Surfaces, San Antonio, TX, USA) is a mechanical valve made entirely of nanosynthesized nitinol, which has been shown in animal models to allow for fast endothelization. The delivery system has also been reduced to a 10-F sheath system, with hopes that this may decrease vascular access site complications.

Further valve technologies such as the ATS 3F series, Lutter Valve, VXi Heart Valve, and Heart Leaflet Technologies Valve combine percutaneous and surgical approaches, and are in their nascent phase of development.

Summary

Transcatheter aortic valve technologies have rapidly evolved in the last decade. Although these advances have clearly laid the groundwork for breakthrough advances, numerous limitations present clinical quandaries that must be overcome before TAVI becomes mainstream. These challenges include development of valves with lower profiles allowing for smaller delivery systems and it is hoped reducing vascular complications. In addition, the development of systems to prevent stroke during or after TAVI implantation, such as filter-based carotid protection devices and the development of valve technologies that decrease the incidence of paravalvular leak while simultaneously decreasing the risk of A-V block and pacemaker requirement, will all be necessary steps in the natural evolution of this potent valvular technology. Nevertheless, although surgery remains the current gold standard for the treatment of aortic valve disease, TAVI is clearly emerging and is poised to settle itself as a niche treatment of patients who cannot undergo SAVR.

PERCUTANEOUS MANAGEMENT OF MITRAL VALVE DISEASE
Background

Mitral valve regurgitation affects approximately 5 million people in the United States and nearly 20 million people worldwide.[1] Primary mitral regurgitation occurs as a result of intrinsic mitral valve disease, resulting from anatomic or congenital changes in the native valve altering its function. This form of mitral regurgitation occurs less frequently than functional mitral regurgitation (FMR), which ensues from left ventricular dilatation and alteration in myocardial geometry. This alteration results in downward displacement of the papillary muscle, leaflet tethering, and annular dilatation. Although surgical repair has been the gold standard of therapy in the modern era for primary mitral regurgitation, the treatment of FMR is less well defined. Surgical therapies for FMR have resulted in high operative morbidity and mortality and significant disease recurrence.[26,27] As a result, patients with symptomatic FMR are often denied surgical therapies.[28] Percutaneous therapies for mitral regurgitation are more complicated than those for aortic stenosis. Reasons for this situation include mitral valve geometry, difficulties with endovascular access, and varying functional properties of different mitral valve pathologies. Essentially, percutaneous mitral valve repair requires treatment of a specific arm of valvular disease, more closely emulating surgery, including indirect annuloplasty, direct ventricular-annular remodeling, and leaflet repair technologies.

Current Status of Transcatheter Mitral Valve Repair

As a result of the complexities of the mitral valve, evolution of percutaneous mitral valve repair has occurred slowly. Surgical techniques have helped to pave the design pathway of novel transcatheter techniques. Although all of the technologies in development have undergone preclinical animal model testing, only a select few have significant human experience, and only 1 technology, the MitraClip Evalve, (Abbott Vascular, Abbott Park, IL, USA) has undergone rigorous testing in a randomized control trial.[8,29] The following sections discuss the current status and future development of percutaneous annuloplasty devices and transcatheter mitral leaflet repair.

Percutaneous Annuloplasty Devices

Annuloplasty is the primary repair mechanism of surgery in patients with FMR. Annular dilation caused by dilation of the left ventricle and distortion of mitral valve geometry is the mechanism of FMR. Although surgical approaches have yet to show clinical benefit in patients with FMR,[30,31] the allure of a percutaneous method of annuloplasty has led to the development of both direct and indirect catheter-based annuloplasty technology.

Current Status of Indirect Annuloplasty

Indirect annuloplasty approaches use the coronary sinus as a route to deliver a device that partially encircles the mitral annulus. Anatomically, the coronary sinus parallels the posterior mitral leaflet, capturing approximately two-thirds of the mitral circumference (**Fig. 2**).[29] Given the already determined feasibility of coronary sinus device implantation, the coronary sinus seemed to be an excellent therapeutic target, and significant interest in this approach spawned the development of at least 3 coronary sinus annuloplasty devices with some human experience: the Cardiac Dimensions Carillon system (Cardiac Dimensions, Kirkland, WA, USA), the Edwards Monarc system (Edwards Lifesciences, Irvine, CA, USA), and the Viacor PTMA system (Viacor, Wilmington,

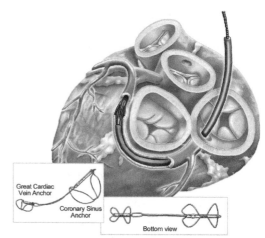

Fig. 2. Coronary sinus annuloplasty using the Carillon mitral annuloplasty device. The coronary sinus encircles at least two-thirds of the mitral annulus, causing it to be an alluring target for indirect annuloplasty devices. The Carillon system uses 2 anchor points and a bridging element that can be positioned in the coronary sinus using a guiding catheter, with final placement creating a shortening effect on the mitral annulus. (*From* Feldman T, Cilingiroglu M. Percutaneous leaflet repair and annuloplasty for mitral regurgitation. J Am Coll Cardiol 2011;57(5):530; with permission.)

MA, USA). Of these 3 systems, only the Cardiac Dimensions Carillon system is still in development.

All of these 3 systems used similar approaches, with transvenous access obtained at the beginning of the case, and implantation of the device in the coronary sinus guided by fluoroscopy. The Carillon system was designed as a simple nitinol wire system engineered into a distal and proximal anchor with a bridging element connecting the 2 systems.[31] On placement in the coronary sinus, the distal anchor is released, and a guiding catheter is used to pull and place tension on the coronary sinus, tightening the mitral annulus and decreasing its circumference. Subsequently the proximal anchor is released, and the device is left in place. With this device, it was possible to decrease mitral regurgitation by at least 1 grade in most patients, with significant improvement in left ventricular volumes and dimensions. Clinically, 6-minute walk tests improved in patients with the device as well, with results remaining for up to 6 months after implantation.[32] With regards to device implantation, this group of devices were successfully implanted in approximately two-thirds of patients, with the remaining one-third undergoing unsuccessful placement as a result of coronary sinus geometry, left circumflex artery compression, or difficult coronary sinus access.[33]

However, long-term durability of the device is questioned, primarily because of the rate of device fracture, which can occur as a result of torsional motion of the coronary sinus during systole.[29] Although device fracture does occur, it is not associated with coronary sinus perforation, and reduction of mitral regurgitation is maintained despite device failure, indicating that sustained positive ventricular remodeling may occur with these annuloplasty devices.[29]

Future Directions for Indirect Annuloplasty Devices

Indirect annuloplasty devices are an attractive approach to the transcatheter treatment of mitral regurgitation. The coronary sinus is a location that has been well studied regarding safety of device implantation, and in addition, the use of transvenous access combined with the general simplicity of the approach allows for these devices to be used in a wide spectrum of patients, including the frail, elderly, and critically ill.

Current limitations of this approach that need to be overcome include overall device stability, which should aim to preclude device fracture and failure. In addition, the ability to avoid left circumflex artery compression currently requires detailed computed tomographic imaging to obtain information regarding the proximity of the coronary sinus to the left circumflex or one of its obtuse marginal branches. The coronary sinus crosses this artery in between two-thirds and three-quarters of patients.[34] Hence, given the nature of this potentially catastrophic event, device manufacturers need to build devices with the ability to be repositioned or retrieved if coronary artery compression occurs acutely.

Current Status of Direct Annuloplasty

A direct annuloplasty device is placed directly into the mitral annulus via a percutaneous guiding catheter similar to a surgical annuloplasty. There are 2 devices in development with limited human experience, namely the Mitralign system (Mitralign, Inc., Tewksbury, MA, USA) and the Guided Delivery Systems device (Guided Delivery Systems, Inc., Santa Clara, CA, USA). Both of these devices obtain a pathway to the posterior mitral annulus through retrograde arterial access via the aortic valve and into the left ventricle. Once positioned, these devices allow a catheter to be positioned near the posterior leaflet. In the Mitralign system, a guide catheter is positioned at the middle scallop of the posterior leaflet, with a radiofrequency (RF) wire used to penetrate the annulus and gain left atrial annular access.

Subsequently, a set of pledgets is deployed in the annulus, and plication with a string draws the mitral circumference closer, shortening it by up to 3 cm. The Guided Delivery Systems device is similar, positioning multiple nitinol-derived anchors into the mitral annulus connected together with a tether, which is drawn back and tensioned. Although these devices have had first-in-human experience, indicating the technical feasibility to the approach, neither long-term nor large-scale data are available with regards to these systems.

Future Directions of Direct Annuloplasty

Although direct annuloplasty is highly anticipated as an alternative approach to surgical annuloplasty and avoids some of the problems in an indirect annuloplasty approach such as coronary sinus geometry limitations and left circumflex artery compression, numerous challenges to this approach continue to exist. First, the approach uses a large-diameter arterial access, adding the risks of vascular site complications to the procedure. In addition, the complexity in delivering such a device in retrograde fashion further adds to difficulty in delivering the device, necessitates a great deal of additional technical training for the operator, and may decrease procedural success. Long-term data in addition to safety and efficacy evaluations in larger patient bases are necessary before direct annuloplasty devices advance clinically.

Percutaneous Leaflet Repair

Surgical leaflet repair is the gold standard treatment of patients with primary mitral regurgitation and generally uses an approach of combining an annuloplasty along with leaflet resection and remodeling. Although leaflet resection is yet to be developed in a percutaneous fashion, transcatheter approaches have primarily focused on emulating a less commonly used surgical technique pioneered by Alfieri and colleagues[35] in the early 1990s. In this technique, named the edge-to-edge repair or the double-orifice repair, the free edges of the mitral leaflets are sutured together to create 2 orifices, effectively narrowing the mitral inflow area and reducing mitral regurgitation. Traditionally, this procedure is performed along with an annuloplasty, although results without an annuloplasty have also had durable clinical outcomes in a small group of patients who were followed for up to 12 years.[36] Thus the concept that this procedure could be replicated percutaneously originated, and the Evalve Mitra-Clip was created.

The Evalve MitraClip uses a small clip deployed via antegrade access from a 24-F transvenous, transseptal catheter approach. This clip is mounted on a delivery system, which is passed through the mitral orifice under echocardiographic guidance. Using a steering system built into the delivery catheter, the clip is positioned anteroposteriorly and mediolaterally. Once positioned at the level of the dysfunctional valve, the clip is opened and closed, and remains in place by the action of small barbs on the inner portion of the clip itself (**Fig. 3**A). While the clip is deployed, fluoroscopic and real-time echocardiographic guidance is obtained (see **Fig. 3**B), and a demonstration of efficacy of mitral regurgitation reduction is seen.[29] If satisfactory positioning is obtained, the clip is deployed; otherwise, repositioning may be performed. In addition, if inadequate mitral regurgitation reduction is noted, an additional clip can be deployed. Patients have been referred for surgical repair after MitraClip deployment, with successful repair having been documented.[37]

Usually, surgical repair after successful clip deployment is performed only for recurrent mitral regurgitation or inadequate reduction of mitral regurgitation. When surgical repair has not been feasible after clip deployment, patients have had other clinical predictors of failed surgical repair including advanced age, annular calcification, and leaflet calcification.[29,37] Hence the confidence engendered by using the clip without altering the possibility of future surgical repair gives immense credit to this burgeoning technology.

The Endovascular Valve Edge-to-Edge Repair Study (EVEREST) II is a phase II randomized clinical trial comparing the MitraClip device against surgical valve repair or replacement. The trial enrolled 279 patients who were randomized in a 2:1 scheme in favor of the percutaneous approach with 1-year and 2-year follow-up. All echocardiographic parameters were assessed at an echocardiographic core laboratory. In this study, the rates of the primary efficacy end point (a composite of freedom from death, from surgery

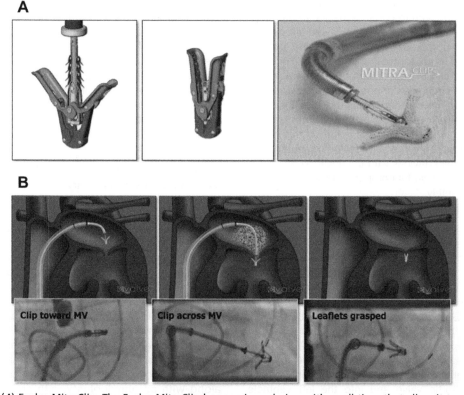

Fig. 3. (*A*) Evalve MitraClip. The Evalve MitraClip has a unique design with small tines that allow it to clasp the mitral leaflets creating a double-orifice similar to the originally described Alfieri surgical approach. (*B*) MitraClip deployment using an antegrade transvenous, transseptal approach. The MitraClip delivery system is advanced from the venous system through a transseptal puncture into the left atrium and left ventricle across the mitral valve. After positioning is confirmed, the device is deployed, and the mitral leaflets are held together by action of the clip. (*From* Feldman T, Cilingiroglu M. Percutaneous leaflet repair and annuloplasty for mitral regurgitation. J Am Coll Cardiol 2011;57(5):533; with permission.)

for valve dysfunction, and from grade 3+ or 4+ mitral regurgitation at 12 months) were 55% in the percutaneous repair group and 73% in the surgery group ($P = .007$).[8] These efficacy end points met the prespecified noninferiority definition. At 2-year follow-up, the proportion of patients with the primary efficacy end point was 52% in the MitraClip group and 66% in the surgery group ($P = .04$).[8] With regards to safety, major adverse events occurred in 15% of patients in the MitraClip group and 48% of patients in the surgery group at 30 days ($P<.001$).[8] This difference was primarily driven by the need for blood transfusions, which has been correlated with a higher rate of mortality when performed after cardiac surgery.[38] In all, a larger proportion of surgery patients had 0 to 1+ mitral regurgitation, but both groups had reductions in left ventricular volumes and dimensions as well as improvements in New York Heart Association functional class.

Future Directions of Percutaneous Leaflet Repair

Although percutaneous leaflet repair seems to be the closest of the percutaneous mitral valve repair strategies to clinical use, numerous limitations still exist. These challenges include a need for long-term data showing sustained benefit in patients. In addition, the EVEREST II trial tested this device primarily in patients with primary mitral regurgitation, whereas registry data after CE Mark approval in Europe has mainly shown use of the device in patients with FMR. The efficacy of the MitraClip in this population is still to be determined. One wonders if the MitraClip strategy may garner further benefit if combined with a percutaneous annuloplasty approach, more closely emulating the original design and success of the Alfieri double-orifice repair.

The Future of Percutaneous Mitral Valve Therapies

Although the development of percutaneous approaches to the treatment of mitral valve disease has lagged behind the development of aortic valve technologies, advances in the last decade have progressed the field to the point of near clinical functionality. Current devices push the boundaries of percutaneous and surgical interventions, and although hampered by limitations, the novel ideas created by these developing systems will create a springboard for further iterative development of these technologies. Future development of RF annuloplasty devices that use RF energy to shrink the mitral annulus, as well as percutaneous mitral valve replacement, are in their nascent phase, only now emerging from preclinical evaluation. Challenges with the mitral valve include its asymmetric shape and lack of a landing zone for anchoring a valve replacement device. The more complex access to the mitral valve also creates technical difficulties, and adjunctive imaging will become even more critical as technologies in this field advance. Although numerous therapeutic ventures have garnered scientific benefit, the lack of funding and economic consequences have halted some promising ideas, including the Coapsys system developed by Myocor. This novel device uses a tether placed through the left ventricular cavity via transpericardial access along with external pads on the anterior and posterior ventricular walls. These pads were then connected with a transventricular cord, meant to compress the ventricle, allowing for

Table 2
Characteristics of an ideal percutaneous valve technology

Aortic Valve Replacement	Mitral Valve Repair
Low profile arterial access	Transvenous access or low profile arterial access
Ability to reposition or retrieve device	Ability to reposition or retrieve device
Delivery system that does not require high level of technical expertise with rapid learning curve	Delivery system that does not require high level of technical expertise with rapid learning curve
Reduction in need for pacemaker implantation	Ability to perform both annuloplasty and leaflet repair
Reduction in stroke risk	Adjunctive intracardiac imaging systems to guide therapeutic procedures
Improved long-term durability of valves	Improved long-term durability of repair
Decrease incidence of paravalvular leaks	Decrease residual mitral regurgitation after percutaneous repair

mitral septal-lateral annular shortening and left ventricular remodeling.

SUMMARY

The transcatheter treatment of cardiac valvulopathies is an emerging field with great promise and a bright future. The therapies being advanced by the pioneers in this field show how ingenuity and novel ideas can translate into direct clinical benefits to the patient. As these therapies are used more in the coming years with further iterations of devices becoming available, and knowledge accrued regarding developing disease, we are certain to see many changes in the fundamental thinking of how we treat patients with complex structural heart disease. The future of percutaneous valve repair and replacement rests in our ability to inch closer to the perfect transcatheter technology (**Table 2**). With continuous tweaks, and countless modifications of current strategies, we hope that we can extend treatment of these diseases to those who previously were not candidates for conventional interventions.

REFERENCES

1. Cubeddu RJ, Palacios IF. Percutaneous heart valve replacement and repair: advances and future potential. Expert Rev Cardiovasc Ther 2009;7(7):811–21.
2. Cubeddu RJ, Jneid H, Don CW, et al. Retrograde versus antegrade percutaneous aortic balloon valvuloplasty: immediate, short- and long-term outcome at 2 years. Catheter Cardiovasc Interv 2009;74(2): 225–31.
3. Kan JS, White RI Jr, Mitchell SE, et al. Percutaneous balloon valvuloplasty: a new method for treating congenital pulmonary-valve stenosis. N Engl J Med 1982;307(9):540–2.
4. Lock JE, Khalilullah M, Shrivastava S, et al. Percutaneous catheter commissurotomy in rheumatic mitral stenosis. N Engl J Med 1985;313(24): 1515–8.
5. Palacios IF, Lock JE, Keane JF, et al. Percutaneous transvenous balloon valvotomy in a patient with severe calcific mitral stenosis. J Am Coll Cardiol 1986;7(6):1416–9.
6. Al Zaibag M, Ribeiro P, Al Kasab S. Percutaneous balloon valvotomy in tricuspid stenosis. Br Heart J 1987;57(1):51–3.
7. Al Kasab S, Ribeiro P, Al Zaibag M. Use of a double balloon technique for percutaneous balloon pulmonary valvotomy in adults. Br Heart J 1987;58(2): 136–41.
8. Feldman T, Foster E, Glower DG, et al. Percutaneous repair or surgery for mitral regurgitation. N Engl J Med 2011;364(15):1395–406.
9. Smith CR, Leon MB, Mack MJ, et al. Transcatheter versus surgical aortic-valve replacement in high-risk patients. N Engl J Med 2011;364(23): 2187–98.
10. Johri AM, Yared K, Durst R, et al. Three-dimensional echocardiography-guided repair of severe paravalvular regurgitation in a bioprosthetic and mechanical mitral valve. Eur J Echocardiogr 2009; 10(4):572–5.
11. Nkomo VT, Gardin JM, Skelton TN, et al. Burden of valvular heart diseases: a population-based study. Lancet 2006;368(9540):1005–11.
12. Leon MB, Smith CR, Mack M, et al. Transcatheter aortic-valve implantation for aortic stenosis in patients who cannot undergo surgery. N Engl J Med 2010;363(17):1597–607.
13. Schwarz F, Baumann P, Manthey J, et al. The effect of aortic valve replacement on survival. Circulation 1982;66(5):1105–10.
14. Murphy ES, Lawson RM, Starr A, et al. Severe aortic stenosis in patients 60 years of age or older: left ventricular function and 10-year survival after valve replacement. Circulation 1981;64(2 Pt 2):II184–8.
15. O'Brien SM, Shahian DM, Filardo G, et al. The Society of Thoracic Surgeons 2008 cardiac surgery risk models: part 2–isolated valve surgery. Ann Thorac Surg 2009;88(Suppl 1):S23–42.
16. Iung B, Cachier A, Baron G, et al. Decision-making in elderly patients with severe aortic stenosis: why are so many denied surgery? Eur Heart J 2005; 26(24):2714–20.
17. Bouma BJ, van Den Brink RB, van Der Meulen JH, et al. To operate or not on elderly patients with aortic stenosis: the decision and its consequences. Heart 1999;82(2):143–8.
18. Cribier A, Savin T, Saoudi N, et al. Percutaneous transluminal valvuloplasty of acquired aortic stenosis in elderly patients: an alternative to valve replacement? Lancet 1986;1(8472):63–7.
19. Otto CM, Mickel MC, Kennedy JW, et al. Three-year outcome after balloon aortic valvuloplasty. Insights into prognosis of valvular aortic stenosis. Circulation 1994;89(2):642–50.
20. Pedersen WR, Van Tassel RA, Pierce TA, et al. Radiation following percutaneous balloon aortic valvuloplasty to prevent restenosis (RADAR pilot trial). Catheter Cardiovasc Interv 2006;68(2):183–92.
21. Thomas M, Schymik G, Walther T, et al. Thirty-day results of the SAPIEN Aortic Bioprosthesis European Outcome (SOURCE) Registry: A European registry of transcatheter aortic valve implantation using the Edwards SAPIEN valve. Circulation 2010;122(1): 62–9.
22. Paniagua D, Condado JA, Besso J, et al. First human case of retrograde transcatheter implantation of an aortic valve prosthesis. Tex Heart Inst J 2005;32(3):393–8.

23. Del Valle-Fernandez R, Ruiz CE. Transcatheter heart valves for the treatment of aortic stenosis: state-of-the-art. Minerva Cardioangiol 2008;56(5):543–56.

24. Low RI, Bolling SF, Yeo KK, et al. Direct flow medical percutaneous aortic valve: proof of concept. EuroIntervention 2008;4(2):256–61.

25. Schofer J, Schluter M, Treede H, et al. Retrograde transarterial implantation of a nonmetallic aortic valve prosthesis in high-surgical-risk patients with severe aortic stenosis: a first-in-man feasibility and safety study. Circ Cardiovasc Interv 2008;1(2):126–33.

26. Grossi EA, Goldberg JD, LaPietra A, et al. Ischemic mitral valve reconstruction and replacement: comparison of long-term survival and complications. J Thorac Cardiovasc Surg 2001;122(6):1107–24.

27. McGee EC, Gillinov AM, Blackstone EH, et al. Recurrent mitral regurgitation after annuloplasty for functional ischemic mitral regurgitation. J Thorac Cardiovasc Surg 2004;128(6):916–24.

28. Hung J, Papakostas L, Tahta SA, et al. Mechanism of recurrent ischemic mitral regurgitation after annuloplasty: continued LV remodeling as a moving target. Circulation 2004;110(11 Suppl 1):II85–90.

29. Feldman T, Cilingiroglu M. Percutaneous leaflet repair and annuloplasty for mitral regurgitation. J Am Coll Cardiol 2011;57(5):529–37.

30. Wu AH, Aaronson KD, Bolling SF, et al. Impact of mitral valve annuloplasty on mortality risk in patients with mitral regurgitation and left ventricular systolic dysfunction. J Am Coll Cardiol 2005;45(3):381–7.

31. Mihaljevic T, Lam BK, Rajeswaran J, et al. Impact of mitral valve annuloplasty combined with revascularization in patients with functional ischemic mitral regurgitation. J Am Coll Cardiol 2007;49(22):2191–201.

32. Webb JG, Harnek J, Munt BI, et al. Percutaneous transvenous mitral annuloplasty: initial human experience with device implantation in the coronary sinus. Circulation 2006;113(6):851–5.

33. Feldman T. Percutaneous mitral valve repair. J Interv Cardiol 2007;20(6):488–94.

34. Tops LF, Van de Veire NR, Schuijf JD, et al. Noninvasive evaluation of coronary sinus anatomy and its relation to the mitral valve annulus: implications for percutaneous mitral annuloplasty. Circulation 2007;115(11):1426–32.

35. Alfieri O, Maisano F, De Bonis M, et al. The double-orifice technique in mitral valve repair: a simple solution for complex problems. J Thorac Cardiovasc Surg 2001;122(4):674–81.

36. Maisano F, Vigano G, Blasio A, et al. Surgical isolated edge-to-edge mitral valve repair without annuloplasty: clinical proof of the principle for an endovascular approach. EuroIntervention 2006;2(2):181–6.

37. Dang NC, Aboodi MS, Sakaguchi T, et al. Surgical revision after percutaneous mitral valve repair with a clip: initial multicenter experience. Ann Thorac Surg 2005;80(6):2338–42.

38. Murphy GJ, Reeves BC, Rogers CA, et al. Increased mortality, postoperative morbidity, and cost after red blood cell transfusion in patients having cardiac surgery. Circulation 2007;116(22):2544–52.

Index

Note: Page numbers of article titles are in **boldface** type.

A

Ablation, of mitral leaflets, 80

Accucinch Annuloplasty system, for mitral regurgitation, 79, 94–95

Accutrak delivery system, for CoreValve Revalving system, 27

Adenosine, in balloon aortic valvuloplasty, 122–123

Age considerations, in mitral stenosis valvuloplasty, 51

AMADEUS (Carillon Mitral Annuloplasty Device European Union Study), 91

Amplatzer Vascular Plug, for perivalvular regurgitation, 97

Anesthesia
  for balloon pulmonary valvuloplasty, 107
  for Edwards SAPIEN device implantation, 16

Angiography, for balloon pulmonary valvuloplasty, 107–108

Annuloplasty, for mitral regurgitation, 78–79, 89–95, 144–145

Antegrade double-balloon valvuloplasty, for rheumatic mitral stenosis, 47–48, 5556

Antibiotics, for balloon valvuloplasty
  mitral stenosis, 46–47
  pulmonary stenosis, 107

Anticoagulants, for balloon valvuloplasty, for rheumatic mitral stenosis, 47

Aorta, direct approach to, for CoreValve device implantation, 32

Aortic regurgitation, periprosthetic, 37–39, 134

Aortic stenosis, **1–9**
  balloon valvuloplasty for. *See* Balloon valvuloplasty, for aortic stenosis.
  economic impact of, 1
  pathology of, 1–4
  restenosis in, 5
  symptoms of, 1
  valve implantation for. *See* Transcatheter aortic valve implantation (TAVI).

Aortic valve
  damage of, in valvuloplasty, 124–125
  predilatation of, in Edwards SAPIEN device implantation, 17–18, 20

Aortic valve area, after balloon valvuloplasty, 5

Aortic valve implantation, transcatheter. *See* Transcatheter aortic valve implantation (TAVI).

Aortography, for Edwards SAPIEN device implantation, 16–17, 20

AorTx device, for aortic stenosis, 143

Apolipoproteins, in aortic stenosis, 3

Arrhythmias
  in aortic balloon valvuloplasty, 134
  in Edwards SAPIEN device implantation, 23

Ascendra delivery system, for Edwards SAPIEN device, 12, 20

Aspirin, for Edwards SAPIEN device implantation, 16, 20

Atherosclerosis, aortic stenosis and, 1–4

Atrial fibrillation
  after Edwards SAPIEN device implantation, 23
  mitral stenosis valvuloplasty with, 51–52, 55

Atrioventricular block, in aortic balloon valvuloplasty, 134

Axillary artery approach, to balloon aortic valvuloplasty, 122

B

Balloon valvuloplasty
  for aortic stenosis, 4–6, **129–137**
    calcific, 4–6
    complications of, 134
    Edwards SAPIEN device for. *See* Edwards SAPIEN device.
    future directions for, 140–143
    in pediatric patients, **121–128**
    indications for, 130–131
    outcome of, 134–135
    patient selection for, 130–131
    procedure for, 131–134
    versus transcatheter aortic valve implantation, **129–137**
  for pulmonary valve stenosis, 104–116
  for rheumatic mitral stenosis, **45–61**
    complications of, 52–53
    emergency performance of, 45
    gender differences in, 58
    in elderly persons, 54–55
    in pregnancy, 58
    mechanism of, 49
    mitral valve area increase after, 49–52
    optimal candidates for, 56
    outcome of, 49, 53–58
    patient selection for, 45–46
    technique of, 46–49
    versus surgical commissurotomy, 57–58

Moving?

Make sure your subscription moves with you!

To notify us of your new address, find your **Clinics Account Number** (located on your mailing label above your name), and contact customer service at:

Email: journalscustomerservice-usa@elsevier.com

800-654-2452 (subscribers in the U.S. & Canada)
314-447-8871 (subscribers outside of the U.S. & Canada)

Fax number: 314-447-8029

**Elsevier Health Sciences Division
Subscription Customer Service
3251 Riverport Lane
Maryland Heights, MO 63043**

*To ensure uninterrupted delivery of your subscription, please notify us at least 4 weeks in advance of move.

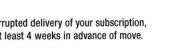

Printed and bound by CPI Group (UK) Ltd, Croydon, CR0 4YY

03/10/2024

01040350-0010